THE USE OF AQUATICS

in Orthopedic and Sports Medicine Rehabilitation and Physical Conditioning

THE USE OF AQUATICS
in Orthopedic and Sports Medicine Rehabilitation and Physical Conditioning

Kevin E. Wilk, PT, DPT, FAPTA
ASSOCIATE CLINICAL DIRECTOR
CHAMPION SPORTS MEDICINE
DIRECTOR OF REHABILITATIVE RESEARCH
AMERICAN SPORTS MEDICINE INSTITUTE
BIRMINGHAM, ALABAMA
REHABILITATION CONSULTANT
TAMPA BAY RAYS BASEBALL ORGANIZATION
TAMPA BAY, FLORIDA

David M. Joyner, MD, FACS
DIRECTOR OF ATHLETICS
THE PENNSYLVANIA STATE UNIVERSITY
UNIVERSITY PARK, PENNSYLVANIA

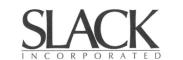

SLACK
INCORPORATED

www.Healio.com/books

ISBN: 978-1-55642-951-4

Copyright © 2014 by SLACK Incorporated

The procedures and practices described in this publication should be implemented in a manner consistent with the professional standards set for the circumstances that apply in each specific situation. Every effort has been made to confirm the accuracy of the information presented and to correctly relate generally accepted practices. The authors, editors, and publisher cannot accept responsibility for errors or exclusions or for the outcome of the material presented herein. There is no expressed or implied warranty of this book or information imparted by it. Care has been taken to ensure that drug selection and dosages are in accordance with currently accepted/recommended practice. Off-label uses of drugs may be discussed. Due to continuing research, changes in government policy and regulations, and various effects of drug reactions and interactions, it is recommended that the reader carefully review all materials and literature provided for each drug, especially those that are new or not frequently used. Some drugs or devices in this publication have clearance for use in a restricted research setting by the Food and Drug and Administration or FDA. Each professional should determine the FDA status of any drug or device prior to use in their practice.

Any review or mention of specific companies or products is not intended as an endorsement by the author or publisher.

SLACK Incorporated uses a review process to evaluate submitted material. Prior to publication, educators or clinicians provide important feedback on the content that we publish. We welcome feedback on this work.

Published by: SLACK Incorporated
                     6900 Grove Road
                     Thorofare, NJ 08086 USA
                     Telephone: 856-848-1000
                     Fax: 856-848-6091
                     www.Healio.com/books

Contact SLACK Incorporated for more information about other books in this field or about the availability of our books from distributors outside the United States.

                 Library of Congress Cataloging-in-Publication Data

The use of aquatics in orthopedic and sports medicine rehabilitation and physical conditioning / [edited by] Kevin E. Wilk and David Joyner.
     p. ; cm.
  Includes bibliographical references and index.
  ISBN 978-1-55642-951-4 (alk. paper)
  I. Wilk, Kevin E., editor of compilation. II. Joyner, David, 1950- editor of compilation.
  [DNLM: 1. Hydrotherapy--methods. 2. Physical Fitness. 3. Rehabilitation--methods. WB 520]
  RM813
  615.8'53--dc23
                     2013019399

For permission to reprint material in another publication, contact SLACK Incorporated. Authorization to photocopy items for internal, personal, or academic use is granted by SLACK Incorporated provided that the appropriate fee is paid directly to Copyright Clearance Center. Prior to photocopying items, please contact the Copyright Clearance Center at 222 Rosewood Drive, Danvers, MA 01923 USA; phone: 978-750-8400; website: www.copyright.com; email: info@copyright.com

Printed in the United States of America.

Last digit is print number: 10   9   8   7   6   5   4   3   2   1

DEDICATION

This textbook is dedicated to my family, my wife Debbie, and children Justin, Summer, and Brittney, who have given me support, encouragement, and energy to continue to pursue my professional goals.

Thanks to all my patients, colleagues, and mentors who I have learned so much from.

Thank you and I hope you enjoy this work.

Kevin E. Wilk, PT, DPT, FAPTA

I would like to dedicate this textbook to my wife Carolyn; my children Andy, Matt, and Kate; and all of my family. They have been unending in their support and loyalty as I have undertaken the many paths of my life. Also to my many patients, teachers, and teammates who have taught me the lessons of life and professional pursuits. My thanks to all.

David M. Joyner, MD, FACS

CONTENTS

ACKNOWLEDGMENTS

I would like to thank Lenny Macrina, MS, PT and Susan McWhorter for their assistance in the editing and preparation of this textbook.

I would like to thank Anson Flake for his energy and efforts in completing this textbook.

Thanks to Carrie Kotlar for her hard work and dedication in completing this textbook.

Kevin E. Wilk, PT, DPT, FAPTA
David M. Joyner, MD, FACS

ABOUT THE EDITORS

Kevin E. Wilk, PT, DPT, FAPTA, has lead a distinguished career as a clinical physical therapist for the past 30 years as a leading authority in rehabilitation of sports injuries and orthopedic lesions. He has made significant contributions to laboratory research, biomechanical research, and clinical outcome studies.

Dr. Wilk has been a physical therapist, researcher, and educator for 30 years. Dr. Wilk is currently Associate Clinical Director for Champion Sports Medicine (a Physiotherapy Facility) in Birmingham, AL. In addition, he is the Director of Rehabilitative Research at the American Sports Medicine Institute in Birmingham and is Adjunct Assistant Professor in the Physical Therapy Program at Marquette University in Milwaukee, WI. Dr. Wilk is also the Rehabilitation Consultant for the Tampa Bay Rays' baseball team, and has worked with the Rays for 16 years. Dr. Wilk has worked with professional baseball for 26 years, and with the Rays since the organization started. Dr. Wilk received his physical therapy degree from Northwestern University Medical School in Chicago, IL, and his DPT from Massachusetts General Hospital Institute of Health Professions in Boston, MA.

Dr. Wilk has published over 155 journal articles, over 98 book chapters, and has lectured at over 700 professional and scientific meetings. Dr. Wilk is on the review boards of 9 journals. Dr. Wilk has received numerous professional awards. In 2012, he was inducted into the Sports Section Blackburn Hall of Fame. Later that same year he was awarded the APTA Catherine Worthingham Fellowship—the highest honor given to an APTA member. Dr. Wilk stated he was humbled and tremendously honored to receive these 2 prestigious recognitions. In 2004, Dr. Wilk received the prestigious Ron Peyton Award for career achievement from the Sports Physical Therapy Section of the APTA. He has received the James Andrews Award for achievement in the area of baseball science. Dr. Wilk was an honored professor at several universities, has given grand rounds at numerous medical facilities, and has lectured internationally. Including this book, he has edited 8 textbooks: *The Athletes' Shoulder* (2nd ed), *Rehabilitation of the Injured Athlete* (3rd ed), *Injuries in Baseball, Sports Medicine of Baseball, Orthopaedic Rehabilitation* (2nd ed), *Handbook of Orthopaedic Rehabilitation* (2nd ed), and *The Orthopaedic Toolbox* (2nd ed).

Dr. Wilk has served as President of the Sports Section of the APTA from June 2007 to June 2010, and has served as Vice President, Education Program Chairman, and Editor of the Home Study Course for the Sports Physical Therapy Section of the APTA for 7 years previously and has served on numerous committees for the APTA. Dr. Wilk was the first nonphysician named to a committee for the American Orthopaedic Society for Sports Medicine (AOSSM).

Dr. Wilk is a clinician, researcher, and educator and is generally regarded as one of the leading sports physical therapist experts in the evaluation and treatment of shoulder, knee, and elbow joint injuries. He is active daily with patient care, research, and educational activities. His seminars are extremely well attended and receive excellent reviews based on scientific evidence, clinical experience, innovative approaches, and his interactive and fun approach to seminars. He is continuously updating and changing his seminars to meet the demands of the ever changing health care environment.

David M. Joyner, MD, FACS, was named Penn State's Acting Director of Athletics on November 16, 2011 and assumed the title of Director of Athletics on January 21, 2012.

A 2-sport All-American and Academic All-American at Penn State, Dr. Joyner earned his bachelor's degree in science in 1972 and his MD from Penn State's College of Medicine in 1976. Following residencies in general and orthopedic surgery at The Milton S. Hershey Medical Center and a stint in the World Football League, Dr. Joyner began a medical career with a sports medicine emphasis.

Dr. Joyner is a health care and business consultant and an orthopedic physician. Founder, Chairman, and CEO of Joyner SportsMedicine Institute (JSI) from 1992 to 1998, he developed 19 physical therapy centers in 8 states to deliver state-of-the-art training and rehabilitation services honed by US Olympic and Elite Medical Team experience and leadership.

Closely involved with numerous campus initiatives, Dr. Joyner has served as a member of Penn State Libraries Development Advisory Board, co-chairman of the Paterno Libraries Endowment, chairman of the external advisory board for the Schreyer Institute for Teaching Excellence and the Schreyer Honors College, a member of the Hershey Medical Center Capital Campaign Committee, and was active in the Grand Destiny Campaign for Athletics. He is a member of the board of directors of The Milton S. Hershey Medical Center.

A member of the Penn State Board of Trustees from 2000 until the date of his appointment with Intercollegiate Athletics, Dr. Joyner was honored in 1992 as a Distinguished Alumnus of Penn State.

Dr. Joyner's work with the US Olympic Committee includes service as head physician to the United States' teams at the 1992 Olympic Winter Games, the 1991 World University Games, and the 1989 United States Olympic Festival. He is a past chairman of the US Olympic Committee Sports Medicine Society. Dr. Joyner served as the chairman of the US Olympic Committee's Sports Medicine Committee and the vice-chairman of the US Olympic Committee's Anti-Doping Committee. He currently is a member of the medical commission of the Pan American Sports Organization.

Dr. Joyner served on the Pennsylvania Governor's Council on Physical Fitness and Sports and is Chairman of USA Football's Football Wellness Committee and has been an emeritus member of the American Orthopedic Society for Sports Medicine.

A Penn State offensive tackle from 1969 to 1971, Dr. Joyner earned first-team All-America honors in his senior season and was a team co-captain. He was instrumental in helping the Nittany Lions earn a cumulative 29-4 record, including an 11-0 mark in 1969, with victories in the 1970 Orange and 1972 Cotton Bowls. Dr. Joyner also was a standout wrestler from 1970 to 1972, earning All-America honors by finishing as the NCAA runner-up at heavyweight in 1971.

Dr. Joyner was named a first-team CoSIDA Academic All-American in 1971 and is one of a select group of individuals who have been inducted into the CoSIDA Academic All-America Hall of Fame, which honors "those with the highest standards in college academics, athletics and in life beyond athletics." Dr. Joyner also earned an NCAA Postgraduate Scholarship as a Penn State student-athlete and was selected for the prestigious NCAA Silver Anniversary Award in 1997.

Dr. Joyner was inducted into the Pennsylvania Sports Hall of Fame in 1994 and the Pennsylvania Wrestling Hall of Fame in 1993.

Dr. Joyner's sons Andy and Matt also played football at Penn State and are graduates of the university.

Contributing Authors

James R. Andrews, MD (Foreword)
American Sports Medicine Institute
Andrews Sports Medicine and Orthopaedic Center
Birmingham, Alabama

Bruce E. Becker, MD, MS, FACSM (Chapter 1)
Director, National Aquatics & Sports Medicine Institute
Washington State University
Clinical Professor
University of Washington School of Medicine
Seattle, Washington

Stephen F. Crouse, PhD, FACSM (Chapter 10)
Professor of Kinesiology
Texas A&M University
College Station, Texas

Timothy DiFrancesco, PT, DPT, ATC, CSCS, AQx, CMT
(Chapter 6)
Head Strength and Conditioning Coach
Los Angeles Lakers
Los Angeles, California

Dennis Dolny, PhD (Chapter 10)
Utah State University
Logan, Utah

Anson J. Flake, Esq (Chapter 3)
CEO and Cofounder
HydroWorx
Middletown, Pennsylvania

Murphy Grant, MS, ATC, NASM-PES, CES
(Chapters 8 and 9)
Assistant Athletic Director–Sports Medicine
University of Kansas
Lawrence, Kansas

Jessica Heath, PT, OCS, Cert MDT, CSCS (Chapter 2)
Clinical Education and Residency Manager
Drayer Physical Therapy Institute
Hummelstown, Pennsylvania

Todd R. Hooks, PT, DMT, OCS, SCS, ATC, MOMT, MTC,
CSCS, FAAOMPT (Chapter 4)
Beacon Orthopaedics and Cincinnati Reds Baseball
  Organization
Cincinnati, Ohio

Leonard C. Macrina, MSPT, SCS, CSCS (Chapter 5)
Champion Sports Medicine
Birmingham, Alabama

Jason Palmer, BHMS (Ed) Hons, BPhty, MCSP (Chapter 4)
Physiotherapist
Chelsea Football Club
London, England

Lisa Pataky, PT, DPT (Chapters 2 and 6)
Star Physical Therapy
New York, New York

Mike Reinold, DPT, ATC, CSCS (Chapter 5)
Consultant
Champion Physical Therapy & Performance
Boston, Massachusetts

Daniel Seidler, PT, MS (Chapter 7)
WSPT Physical Therapy
Bronx, New York

A. J. Yenchak, PT, DPT, CSCS (Chapter 5)
Columbia Sports Therapy
Columbia Doctors Midtown
New York, New York

FOREWORD

This book is a very important step forward in the sports medicine field and has the potential of taking aquatic rehabilitation to a whole new level.

As evidenced in this book, aquatic rehabilitation and exercise has come a long way from traditional swimming pool therapy 20 years ago to specialized aquatic exercise pools with treadmills, resistance jets, video cameras, and exercise equipment in today's modern sports medicine world.

This book represents a new generation of rehabilitation that is informative enough to be injury and sports specific. For many years it has been known that protecting joint surfaces and yet being able to rehabilitate articular cartilage is complicated and can be done underwater without fear of impact loading. Aquatic rehabilitation is also therefore important because it allows gradual progressive loading of major joints by specifics, which is well outlined in this book. The end result is allowing joints to have immediate full range of motion with less joint loading.

This book has 10 chapters discussing all parameters of aquatic rehabilitation. The contents covers the history of aquatic rehabilitation all the way through to setup and design to specific rehab exercises and concepts. The 10 chapters include chapters on the upper and lower extremities, spine, chronic pain, and fibromyalgia, including training and conditioning. There is even a chapter on research and its effects on the advancement of aquatic exercises.

The appendix includes 10 specific protocols for various lesions and disorders. As stated above, these protocols can be injury specific as well as sports specific. Some 15 contributors and authors from all over the world with various backgrounds have lent their expertise to this wonderful work of aquatic knowledge.

In summary, this book is a welcome addition to the library of physical therapists, athletic trainers, strength and conditioning coaches, personal trainers, and sports medicine physicians at all levels as well as coaches. It is hoped that it will initiate a new era in the use and development of aquatic therapy in sports medicine rehabilitation.

James R. Andrews, MD
American Sports Medicine Institute
Andrews Sports Medicine and Orthopaedic Center
Birmingham, Alabama

INTRODUCTION

"It's what you learn after you know it all that counts most."
Coach John Wooden

The use of aquatic exercise and hydrotherapy has been utilized for well over 100 years. In 1910, the Spaulding School for Crippled Children in Chicago utilized wooden tanks for paralyzed patients to exercise in.[1] Furthermore, therapeutic tubs were used to treat cerebral palsy patients across the country; one such place was the Orthopaedic Hospital in Los Angeles (which later became Rancho Los Amigos) under the direction of Dr. Charles Leroy Lowman.[1] Leroy Hubbard treated Franklin Roosevelt in Warm Springs, Georgia with his famous aquatic tank. During the 1930s in Hot Springs, Arkansas warm swimming pools were installed, this provided an environment for aquatic exercises and physical therapy in the water.[2] By 1937, Dr. Charles Leroy Lowman published his *Technique of Underwater Gymnastics: A Study in Practical Application*, in which he detailed aquatic therapy methods for specific underwater exercises that "carefully regulated dosage, character, frequency, and duration for remedying bodily deformities and restoring muscle function."[3] Thus, as you can clearly see aquatic therapy and exercise has a long history but has significantly advanced to a sophisticated level since its early days. Today, aquatic exercise pools have underwater treadmills, underwater video cameras, numerous aquatic exercise equipment pieces, and highly skilled aquatic therapists.

The use of aquatic exercises and therapy has been used in the care of high level athletes during their rehabilitation progress back to competition and to provide an effective environment for performance training. These athletes include Bo Jackson, Carson Palmer, Adrian Peterson, Robert Griffin III, Tiger Woods, Derek Jeter, Wilt Chamberlain, Mo Farah, Gail Devers, Florence Griffith-Joyner, and Galen Rupp.

The purpose of this book is to explain the unique benefits of aquatic exercise. Furthermore, we explore the physiologic effects of aquatic exercises, describe and discuss specific exercises for various pathologies, and discuss how the pool can be altered (water temperature, depth, resistance, applied equipment, etc) to obtain the most beneficial effects for the patients. In this book we discuss numerous pathologies and lesions.

The textbook is set up in 5 sections for easy reference and reading. Each chapter is written by experts in the field of aquatic exercise. In Section I, the authors provide the reader with background historical information regarding aquatic rehabilitation and exercise and how to pick and design a pool for your facility. In Section II, the authors discuss specific treatment interventions and treatments for specific lesions of the lower extremity, upper extremity, spine, and chronic pain patients. The next section discusses concepts of strength and conditioning and sports-specific training techniques. Section IV describes the evidence supporting aquatic training and discusses the current research in aquatic exercise and conditioning. The last section of the book are appendices, which offer the reader various treatment protocols, exercise concepts, and specific drills to assist in making this information practical and useful.

It is the hope of the people involved in this book that aquatic exercise becomes a part of every patient's rehabilitation program and becomes part of training for numerous athletes when conditioning for fitness or competitive events.

We hope this book helps the reader in developing and applying the wonderful benefits of aquatic exercise and therapy in their daily practice.

Kevin E. Wilk, PT, DPT, FAPTA
David M. Joyner, MD, FACS

REFERENCES

1. Becker BE. Aquatic therapy: scientific foundations and clinical rehabilitation applications. *PM R.* 2009;1(9):859-872.
2. deVierville J. A history of aquatic rehabilitation. In: Cole A, Becker B, eds. *Comprehensive Aquatic Rehabilitation.* 2nd ed. Philadelphia, PA: Butterworth-Heinemann; 2004:1-18.
3. Lowman CL. *Technique of Underwater Gymnastics: A Study in Practical Application.* Los Angeles, CA: American Publications; 1937.

Section I

Pre-Use and Preparation

Aquatic Therapy
History, Theory, and Applications

Bruce E. Becker, MD, MS, FACSM

Since the earliest recorded history, water has been believed to promote healing and has therefore been widely used in the management of medical ailments. Through observation and centuries of trial and error and scientific methodology, traditions of healing through aquatic treatments have evolved. This review will detail the current scientific understanding of the profound physiologic changes that occur during aquatic immersion. Aquatic immersion has profound biologic effects, extending across essentially all homeostatic systems. These effects are both immediate and delayed, and they allow water to be used with therapeutic efficacy for a great variety of rehabilitative problems. Aquatic therapies are beneficial in the management of patients with musculoskeletal problems, neurologic problems, cardiopulmonary pathology, and other conditions. In addition, the margin of therapeutic safety is wider than that of almost any other treatment milieu. Knowledge of these biological effects can aid the skilled clinician in creating an optimal treatment plan through appropriate modification of aquatic activities, immersion temperatures, and treatment duration.

THE HISTORY OF HYDROTHERAPY

Historically both in Europe and in the Americas, hydrotherapy has been used as a central treatment methodology in recovery from injury and chronic disease. Throughout all recorded history, the sick and suffering have resorted to springs, baths, and pools for their soothing, healing, and powerful effects. "Taking the waters," soaking in baths and pools, and resting at places called spas played an important social and spiritual role in the river valley civilizations of Mesopotamia, Egypt, India, and China. Ritual bathing pools were widely used for individual and social renewal and healing. Healing water rituals also appeared in ancient Greek, Hebrew, Roman, Christian, and Islamic cultures.[1] During the Middle Ages in Europe, the emergence of formal resorts formed for the purposes of healing. These became the progenitors of the current group of European spas. In 1911, Dr. Charles Leroy Lowman, the founder of the Orthopaedic Hospital in Los Angeles, which later became Rancho Los Amigos, began using therapeutic tubs to treat spastic patients and those with cerebral palsy after a visit to the Spaulding School for Crippled Children in Chicago, where he observed paralyzed patients exercising in a wooden tank. On returning to California, he transformed the hospital's lily pond into 2 therapeutic pools.[1] At Warm Springs, Georgia, Leroy Hubbard developed his famous tank, and in 1924 Warm Springs received its most famous aquatic patient, Franklin D. Roosevelt. A wealth of information, research, and articles on spa therapy and pool treatments appeared in professional journals during the 1930s. At Hot Springs, Arkansas, a warm swimming pool was installed for special underwater physical therapy exercises and pool therapy treatments with chronic arthritic patients.[2] By 1937, Dr. Charles Leroy Lowman published his *Technique of Underwater Gymnastics: A Study in Practical Application*, in which he detailed pool therapy methods of specific underwater exercises that "Specific underwater exercise prescriptions, carefully regulated as to dosage, character, frequency, and duration, are of direct value in the remedying of bodily deformities and the restoration of function."[3(p14-15)] During the 1950s, the National

Wilk KE, Joyner DM. *The Use of Aquatics in Orthopedic and Sports Medicine Rehabilitation and Physical Conditioning* (pp 3-16).

Foundation for Infantile Paralysis supported the corrective swimming pools and hydrogymnastics of Dr. Charles Leroy Lowman and the therapeutic use of pools and tanks for the treatment of poliomyelitis.[4] With the advent of polio vaccines and disease-modifying drugs for arthritis, many hospitals filled in their hydrotherapy pools, therapists were no longer trained in aquatic techniques, and the use of hydrotherapy went into a decline. Only since the early 1990s has the use of aquatic therapies dramatically expanded, as recognition of the efficacy and safety of aquatic therapies became widespread among both therapists and medical practitioners. This resurgence is welcome yet reflects a historical legacy. Simon Baruch, the physician father of Bernard Baruch, in 1900 wrote in the Preface to the second edition of *The Principles and Practice of Hydrotherapy*, "So flexible is this therapeutic agent that, unlike medicinal remedies, it may be utilized to meet indications which seem contradictory to the uninitiated."[5] This statement holds true today.

THE PHYSICAL PRINCIPLES OF WATER

Nearly all of the biological effects of immersion are related to the fundamental principles of hydrodynamics. I will briefly describe these principles to make the medical application process more rational. The essential physical properties of water that effect physiologic change are density, specific gravity, hydrostatic pressure, buoyancy, viscosity, and thermodynamics.

Although the human body is mostly water, the body's density is slightly less than that of water and averages a specific gravity of 0.974, with males averaging higher densities than females. Lean body mass, which includes bone, muscle, connective tissue, and organs, has a typical density near 1.1, whereas fat mass, which includes both essential body fat plus fat in excess of essential needs, has a density of about 0.9.[6] Highly fit and muscular males tend toward specific gravities greater than 1, whereas an unfit or obese male might have a considerably lower specific gravity. Consequently, the human body displaces a volume of water weighing slightly more than the body, forcing the body upward by a force equal to the volume of the water displaced.

Pressure is directly proportional to both the liquid density and the immersion depth when the fluid is incompressible, as water is at the depths used in therapeutic environments. Water exerts a pressure of 22.4 mm Hg/ft of water depth, which translates to 1 mm Hg/1.36 cm (0.54 in.) of water depth. Thus, a human body immersed to a depth of 48 in is subjected to a force equal to 88.9 mm Hg, slightly greater than normal diastolic blood pressure. This is the force that aids the resolution of edema in an injured body part.

Pressure in a fluid increases with depth. A human with specific gravity of 0.97 reaches floating equilibrium when 97% of his or her volume is submerged. As the body is gradually immersed, water is displaced, creating the force of buoyancy. This takes the weight off the immersed joints progressively, and with neck immersion, only about 15 lb of compressive force (the approximate weight of the head) is exerted on the spine, hips, and knees. A person immersed to the symphysis pubis has effectively off-loaded 40% of his or her body weight, and when further immersed to the umbilicus, approximately 50% of body weight is off-loaded. Xyphoid immersion off-loads body weight by 60% or more, depending on whether the arms are overhead or beside the trunk.[7] A body suspended or floating in water essentially counterbalances the downward effects of gravity with the upward force of buoyancy. This effect may be of great therapeutic utility. For example, a fractured pelvis may not become mechanically stable under full body loading for a period of 8 to 12 weeks, but with water immersion, gravitational forces may be partially or completely offset so that only muscle torque forces act on the fracture site, allowing active-assisted range-of-motion activities, gentle strength building, and even gait training.

Viscosity refers to the magnitude of internal friction specific to a fluid during motion. When a limb moves relative to water, it is subjected to the resistive effects of the fluid, called drag force, and is due to fluid viscosity and turbulence when present. Under turbulent flow conditions, this resistance increases as a log function of velocity and depends on the shape and size of the object. Although the greatest surface area drag in a swimming person is the head, the negative pressure following the swimmer causes the greatest force resisting forward movement. Viscosity is a quality that makes water a useful strengthening medium. Viscous resistance increases as more force is exerted against it. The power to overcome drag resistance under turbulent conditions increases as the cube of velocity; thus, doubling the speed of an arm moving through water requires 8 times (2^3) the power.[8] That resistance drops to zero almost immediately on cessation of force because there is only a small amount of inertial moment because viscosity effectively counteracts inertial momentum. Thus, when a rehabilitating person feels pain and stops movement, the force drops precipitously and water viscosity damps movement almost instantaneously. This allows great control of strengthening activities within the envelope of patient comfort.[9]

THERMODYNAMICS

Water retains 1000 times more heat than an equivalent volume of air does. The therapeutic utility of water depends greatly on both its ability to retain heat and its ability to transfer heat energy. Water is an efficient conductor, transferring heat 25 times faster than air.[8] This thermal conductive property, in combination with the high specific heat of water, makes the use of water in rehabilitation very versatile because water retains heat or cold while easily delivering it to the immersed body part. Table 1-1 details appropriate temperatures for various aquatic activities.

Table 1-1.

Aquatic Temperatures and Appropriate Activities

Suitable Activities	Cold (10°C to 15°C)	Cool (26°C to 29°C)	Neutral (33.5°C to 35.5°C)	Warm (36°C to 38.5°C)
Postexertional recovery	+			
Contrast baths	+			+
Vigorous exercise		+		
Arthritis exercise			+	
Typical aquatic therapy			+	
Cardiac rehab			+	
Multiple sclerosis exercise		+		
SCI programs			+	
Parkinson's programming			+	
Relaxation				+

These physical effects start immediately on immersion. Heat transfer begins, and because the specific heat of the human body is less than that of water, the body equilibrates faster than water does. Hydrostatic pressure effects begin immediately, although most of these effects are to cause plastic deformation of the body through time (for example, blood displaces cephalad, right atrial pressure begins to rise, pleural surface pressure rises, the chest wall compresses, and the diaphragm is displaced cephalad).

APPLICATIONS IN CARDIOVASCULAR AND CARDIOPULMONARY REHABILITATION

Because an individual immersed in water is subjected to external water pressure in a gradient, which within a relatively small depth exceeds venous pressure, blood is displaced upward through the venous and lymphatic systems, first into the thighs, then into the abdominal cavity vessels, and finally into the great vessels of the chest cavity and into the heart. Central venous pressure rises with immersion to the xyphoid and increases until the body is completely immersed.[10] There is an increase in pulse pressure as a result of the increased cardiac filling and decreased heart rate during thermoneutral immersion.[11,12] Pulmonary blood flow increases with increased central blood volume and pressure. Most of the increased pulmonary blood volume is distributed in the larger vessels of the pulmonary vascular bed, and only a small percentage (≤5%) is at the capillary level.[13] Central blood volume increases by approximately 0.7 L during immersion to the neck, a 60% increase in central volume, with one third of this volume taken

up by the heart and the remainder by the great vessels of the lungs.[10] Cardiac volume increases 27% to 30% with immersion to the neck.[14] Stroke volume increases as a result of this increased stretch. Although normal resting stroke volume is about 71 mL/beat, the additional 25 mL resulting from immersion equals about 100 mL, which is close to the exercise maximum for a sedentary deconditioned individual on land with both an increase in end-diastolic volume and a decrease in end-systolic volume.[15] Mean stroke volume thus increases 35% on average during neck depth immersion even at rest. As cardiac filling and stroke volume increase with progress in immersion depth from symphysis to xyphoid, the heart rate typically drops and typically at average pool temperatures the rate lowers by 12% to 15%.[16,17] This drop is variable, with the amount of decrease dependent on water temperature. (Figure 1-1 depicts these changes.) In warm water, the heart rate generally rises significantly, contributing to yet a further rise in cardiac output at high temperatures.[18,19]

In deep water running, oxygen consumption (VO_2) is 3 times greater at a given speed of running (53 m/min) in water than on land.[20] Thus, looking at the reverse effect, during water walking and running, only one half to one third the speed is required to achieve the same metabolic intensity as on land.[21] The relationship of heart rate to VO_2 during water exercise parallels that of land-based exercise, though water heart rate averages 10 bpm less, for reasons discussed.[10] Consequently, metabolic intensity in water, as on land, may be predicted from monitoring the heart rate.

Cardiac output increases by about 1500 mL/min during clavicle depth immersion, of which 50% is directed to increased muscle blood flow.[16] Because immersion to this depth produces a cardiac stroke volume of about 100 mL/beat, a resting pulse of 86 bpm produces a cardiac output of 8.6 L/min and is already producing cardiac

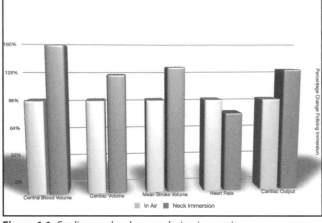

Figure 1-1. Cardiovascular changes during immersion.

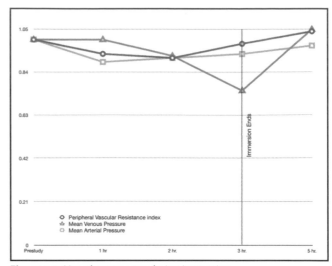

Figure 1-2. Vascular pressures during immersion.

exercise. The increase in cardiac output appears to be somewhat age dependent, with younger subjects demonstrating greater increases (up 59%) than older subjects (up only 22%) and is also highly temperature dependent, varying directly with temperature increase, from 30% at 33°C to 121% at 39°C.[19,22] In general, research has shown aquatic exercise to be at least the equivalent in training value to land-based training, which may refute the myth that water exercise is not an aerobically efficient training method.[23–27]

During immersion to the neck, decreased sympathetic vasoconstriction reduces both peripheral venous tone and systemic vascular resistance by 30% at thermoneutral temperatures, dropping during the first hour of immersion and lasting for a period of hours thereafter.[10] This decreases end-diastolic pressures. Systolic blood pressure increases with increasing workload but generally is approximately 20% lower in water than on land.[19] Most studies show either no change in mean blood pressure or a drop in pressures during immersion in normal pool temperatures (Figure 1-2). Sodium-sensitive hypertensive patients have been noted to show even greater drops (–18 to –20 mm Hg) than normotensive patients, and sodium-insensitive patients show smaller drops (–5 to –14 mm Hg).[28] Studies done in our laboratory demonstrated concurrence with these findings, with systolic and diastolic pressure decreases seen in cool, neutral, and warm water immersion in both young and older populations.[29,30] Based on a substantial body of research, the therapeutic pool appears to be a safe and potentially therapeutic environment for both normotensive and hypertensive patients, in contrast to widespread belief.

Recent research has generally supported the use of aquatic environments in cardiovascular rehabilitation following infarct and ischemic cardiomyopathy. Japanese investigators studied patients with severe congestive heart failure (ejection fraction means 25 ± 9%), under the hypothesis that in this clinical problem, the essential pathology was the inability of the heart to overcome peripheral vascular resistance. They reasoned that because exposure to a warm environment causes peripheral vasodilatation, a reduction in vascular resistance and cardiac afterload might be

therapeutic. During a series of studies, these researchers found that during a single 10-min immersion in a hot water bath, both pulmonary wedge pressure and right atrial pressure dropped by 25%, whereas cardiac output and stroke volume both increased. In a subsequent study of patients using warm water immersion or sauna bath 1 to 2 times per day, 5 days a week for 4 weeks, they found improvement in ejection fractions of nearly 30% along with reduction in left ventricular end-diastolic dimension, along with subjective improvement in quality of life, sleep quality and general well-being.[31] Studies of elderly individuals with systolic congestive heart failure during warm water immersion found that most of these individuals demonstrated an increase in cardiac output and ejection fractions during immersion.[32,33] Caution is prudent when working with individuals with severe valvular insufficiency, because cardiac enlargement may mechanically worsen this problem during full immersion. A Swiss researcher studied individuals with more severe heart failure and concluded that aquatic therapy is probably not safe for individuals with very severe or uncontrolled failure or very recent myocardial infarction.[34–36] That said, a recent summary of published research in this areas has concluded that aquatic and thermal therapies may be a very useful rehabilitative technique in individuals with mild to moderate heart failure.[37]

APPLICATIONS IN MUSCULOSKELETAL REHABILITATION

Water immersion causes significant effects on the musculoskeletal system as well. The effects are caused by the compressive effects of immersion as well as reflex regulation of blood vessel tone. During immersion, it is likely that most of the increased cardiac output is redistributed to skin and muscle rather than to the splanchnic beds.[38] Resting muscle blood flow has been found to increase from a dry baseline

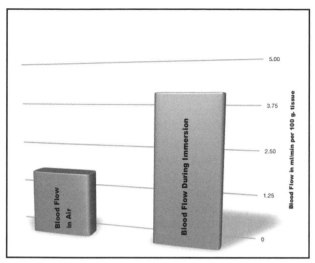

Figure 1-3. Muscle blood flow during immersion.

of 1.8 mL/min/100 g tissue to 4.1 mL/min/100 g tissue with neck immersion with muscle blood flow increased 225% above dry land flow, even higher than the rise in cardiac output during immersion; it is reasonable to conclude that oxygen delivery is significantly increased during immersion at rest[39] (Figure 1-3). Blood flow during exercise is likely enhanced as well and there is research that supports this supposition, finding a 20% increase in blood flow in sedentary middle-aged subjects subjected to 12 weeks of swim training.[40] The hydrostatic effects of immersion, possibly combined with temperature effects, have been shown to significantly improve dependent edema and subjective pain symptoms in patients with venous varicosities.[41] Similarly, a rehabilitation program of hydrotherapy using contrasting temperatures produced subjective improvement, systolic blood pressure increases in the extremities, and significant increases in ambulation in patients with intermittent claudication.[23,24,27,42,43]

APPLICATIONS IN OSTEOARTHRITIS AND INFLAMMATORY ARTHRITIS

The buoyancy of water combined with the hydrostatic pressure produced during immersion and the thermal properties of water make the aquatic environment uniquely beneficial in the management of patients with osteoarthritis. Aquatic therapy has shown to be effective in reducing pain and stiffness and producing high rates of compliance with therapy.[44-49] No studies to date have conclusively demonstrated clear evidence of dramatic differences between land-based and aquatic therapy, although the referenced studies all reported higher rates of subjective gains within the aquatic study groups. In both juvenile and adult rheumatoid arthritis, benefits have been shown from aquatic exercise in symptom reduction, joint mobility, and activities of daily living (ADL) function.[50-56] Most studies

have also demonstrated a subject preference for aquatic versus land exercises, with fewer adverse effects of exercise during aquatic programs.

APPLICATIONS IN ATHLETIC TRAINING

There is a substantial volume of literature that supports the potential value of using aquatic exercise as a cross-training mode.[57-63] It does need to be recognized that though aquatic cross training can present a very significant aerobic challenge to the athlete, there are differences in motor activity, muscle recruitment, and cardiovascular performance.[26,64-68] Though there are some significant differences in cardiovascular function, the overall cardiac demand appears to be at least equivalent.[23,24,27] For maintenance of cardiorespiratory conditioning in highly fit individuals, water running equals dry land running in its effect on maintenance of maximum VO_2 when training intensities and frequencies are matched.[69-71] Similarly, when aquatic exercise is compared with land-based equivalent exercise with regard to the effect on maximum VO_2 gains in unfit individuals, aquatic exercise is seen to achieve equivalent results, and when water temperature is low, the gains achieved are accompanied by a lower heart rate.[72] Thus, water-based exercise programs may be used effectively to sustain or increase aerobic conditioning in athletes who need to keep weight off a joint, as when recovering from injury or during an intensive training program in which joint or bone microtrauma might occur. A key question frequently raised is whether aquatic exercise programs have sufficient specificity to provide a reasonable training venue for athletes in this situation. A study by Kilgore and coworkers specifically addressed the issue of running kinematics during deep water running compared to treadmill running and found a very close comparison between the two when using a cross-country running pattern with respect to knee and ankle kinematics, whereas high-kick running styles did not match the treadmill kinematics.[73] Studies made of aquatic training for plyometric performance have found performance improvement comparable to that of land plyometric training but with reduced posttraining muscle soreness and, of course, decreased joint loading.[74,75] It is unlikely that aquatic training can substantially improve dry land performance in coordination skills such as hurdles, high jump, or other complex coordination activities, where reflex timing becomes a major part of the performance success. But for many athletic activities, aquatic cross-training can sustain or even build aerobic fitness, with the side benefits of reduced joint loading, decreased muscle soreness, and improved performance and a significant potential for improved respiratory function. A study comparing the effects of aggressive resistive exercise in water and on land demonstrated absence of creatine kinase serum levels (an indirect marker of muscle injury) postexercise in the water group, whereas the land group showed near doubled levels.[76] An aquatic exercise program may be designed to

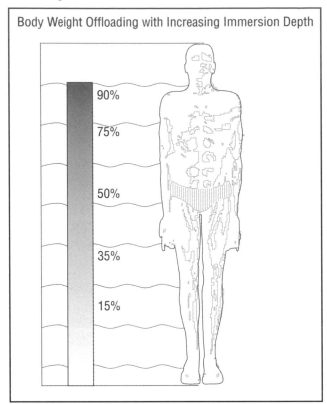

Body Weight Offloading with Increasing Immersion Depth

90%

75%

50%

35%

15%

Figure 1-4. Buoyancy off-loading.

vary the amount of gravity loading by using buoyancy as a counterforce. Rehabilitative programs for specific joints may be more effective as either closed or open kinetic chain programs. Shallow water vertical exercises generally approximate closed-chain exercise, albeit with reduced joint loading because of the counterforce produced by buoyancy. Deep water exercises more generally approximate an open chain system, as do horizontal exercises, such as swimming. Paddles and other resistive equipment tend to close the kinetic chain. Aquatic programs, however, offer the ability to damp the force of movement instantaneously because of the viscous properties of water.

Applications in the Management of Spine Pain

Off-loading of body weight occurs as a function of immersion, but the water depth chosen may be adjusted for the amount of loading desired[7] (Figure 1-4). The spine is especially well protected during aquatic exercise programs, which facilitates early rehabilitation from back injuries. Both clinical experience and comparative literature support active aquatic exercise strategies in spine pain rehabilitation.[77–82] Recent literature has emphasized the benefits of initial nonoperative treatment approaches, and though the role of early surgery remains controversial, most clinical practice revolves around an early trial of therapy. It is in this stage that aquatics may be the most beneficial; as

buoyancy permits offloading, pain is reduced secondary to both afferent nociceptive and thermosensitive inputs, and compliance is usually high.

Spinal stenosis is an unusually vexing problem to the orthopedist and rehabilitation physician, because surgical management is fraught with potential risks. The creation of a conservative management program is also difficult, because often exercise produces symptom aggravation. There does not appear to be any published literature assessing the benefits of aquatic therapy in the conservative management of lumbar spinal stenosis (LSS). The author has had a series of quite dramatic successes in both acquired and congenital LSS, initiating with a nonweight-bearing approach using waist flotation, progressing from a walking to cross-country skiing movement pattern into slow running followed by more active running and gentle lumbar torque movements. One of the most dramatic, a former NFL All-Pro lineman, 6 ft 6 in, weighing 350 lb had advanced multilevel (T11-L5) degenerative LSS, significant electromyographic (EMG) abnormalities at all levels, and severe incapacitation. He underwent an active supervised aquatic rehabilitative program for 6 weeks, with significant functional and symptomatic improvement. He subsequently returned to his ranch in eastern Oregon where he used a backhoe to dig a hole for a plastic septic tank, which he plumbed and filled with warm water to continue his therapy, and for many years the author received annual Christmas cards enthusiastically demonstrating his continued aquatic use.

Respiratory Function in Athletic Rehabilitation

The pulmonary system is profoundly affected by immersion of the body to the level of the thorax. Part of the effect is due to shifting of blood into the chest cavity, and part is due to compression of the chest wall itself by water. The combined effect is to alter pulmonary function, increase the work of breathing, and change respiratory dynamics. Vital capacity decreases about 6% to 9% when comparing neck submersion to controls submerged to the xyphoid with about half reduction due to increased thoracic blood volume and half due to hydrostatic forces counteracting the inspiratory musculature.[83,84] The combined effect of all of these changes is to increase the total work of breathing when submerged to the neck. The total work of breathing at rest for a tidal volume of 1 L increases by 60% during submersion to the neck (Figure 1-5). Of this increased effort, three fourths is attributable to redistribution of blood from the thorax and the rest to increased airway resistance and increased hydrostatic force on the thorax.[83,85–87] Most of the increased work occurs during inspiration. Inspiratory muscle weakness is an important component of many chronic diseases, including congestive heart failure and chronic obstructive lung disease.[88] Because viscosity and flow rates under turbulent conditions enter into the elastic

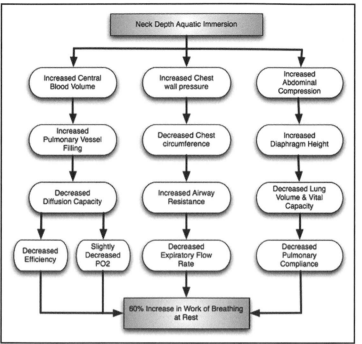

Figure 1-5. Respiratory workload.

workload component of breathing and perhaps into the dynamic component as respiratory rate increases, there is an exponential workload increase with more rapid breathing, as during high-level exercise with rapid respiratory rates.

The combination of respiratory changes makes for a significantly challenging respiratory training environment, especially as respiratory rates increase during high-intensity exercise. Thus, for an athlete used to land-based conditioning exercises, a program of water-based exercise results in a significant workload demand upon the respiratory apparatus, primarily in the muscles of inspiration.[87] Because inspiratory muscle fatigue seems to be a rate- and performance-limiting factor even in highly trained athletes, inspiratory muscle strengthening exercises have proven to be effective in improving athletic performance in elite cyclists and rowers.[89-110] The challenge of inspiratory resistance posed during neck-depth immersion could theoretically raise the respiratory muscular strength and endurance if the time spent in aquatic conditioning is sufficient in intensity and duration to achieve respiratory apparatus strength gains. This theory is supported by research finding that competitive female swimmers adding inspiratory training to conventional swim training realized no improvement in inspiratory endurance compared to the conventional swim-trained controls.[111] These results have been confirmed by more recent studies at the University of Indiana and the University of Toronto.[112,113] The author has had a number of elite athletes comment upon this phenomenon when returning to land-based competition after a period of intense water-based aquatic rehabilitation sufficient to strengthen the respiratory musculature. The common response is a perception of easier breathing at peak exercise levels, effects similar to the studies quoted in elite cyclists and cyclists. This is not surprising in view of the data existing on competitive swimmers who routinely train in the aquatic environment.[111-119] Comparative studies of young swimmers have consistently shown a larger lung capacity (both vital capacity and total lung capacity) and improved forced expiratory capacity, and a number of studies have also shown improvement in inspiratory capacity.[111-113,115,117,119-124]

Respiratory strengthening may be an important aspect of high-level athletic performance, as demonstrated in some of the studies above. When an athlete begins to experience respiratory fatigue, a cascade of physiologic changes follows. The production of metabolites, plus neurologic signaling through the sympathetic nervous system, sends a message to the peripheral arterial tree to shunt blood from the locomotor musculature.[89,125-127] With a decline in perfusion of the muscles of locomotion, the rate of fatigue increases quite dramatically.[90,126] A considerable body of literature supports the plasticity of the respiratory musculature to strengthening with appropriately designed exercise in various disease conditions, although not specifically through aquatic activity.[92,106,108,109,113,128-133] Respiratory muscle weakness, especially in the musculature of inspiration, has been found in chronic heart failure patients, and this weakness is correlated closely with cardiac function and this respiratory weakness may be a significant factor in the impaired exercise capacity seen in individuals with congestive heart failure.[134-138] Because the added work of respiration during immersion occurs almost entirely during the inspiratory phase, it is intriguing to question whether a period of inspiratory muscle strengthening through immersed activity might improve exercise capacity in these individuals.

Aquatic therapy can be useful in the management of patients with neuromuscular impairment of the respiratory system, such as that seen in spinal cord injury and muscular dystrophy.[139–142] A lengthy study of swimming training on cardiorespiratory fitness in spinal cord-injured individuals was done in the late 1970s in Poland. The authors found more than a 440% increase in fitness levels, as contrasted with a 75% increase seen in patients following spinal cord injury in a standard land-based training program over the same period of time.[143] A review in 2006 concluded that respiratory muscle training tended to improve expiratory muscle strength, vital capacity, and residual volume in individuals with spinal cord injury but that insufficient data were available to make conclusions concerning the effects on inspiratory muscle strength, respiratory muscle endurance, quality of life, exercise performance, and respiratory complications.[144]

APPLICATIONS IN GERIATRIC AND OSTEOPOROSIS REHABILITATION

Aquatic exercise has been successfully used to improve balance and coordination in older individuals, who face an increased risk of falling. A 2008 study assessed different forms of aquatic exercise in a group of older subjects and found that deep water running had statistical advantage over typical chest-depth aquatic exercise in reducing balance sway distance and that both exercise forms improved reaction times and movement speed.[145] The hypothesis was that an open-chain exercise such as a deep water program would add an additional balance challenge to the closed-chain exercises typically done. An earlier study assessing aquatic exercise in people with lower extremity arthritis found statistically significant reductions of 18% to 30% in postural sway following 6 weeks of closed-chain training.[146] It may be concluded that both open- and closed-chain exercise in the aquatic environment can produce significant gains in balance, with some evidence that the former adds increased challenge.

Because aquatic exercise, whether through swimming or vertical water exercise, is either limited or nonweight bearing, the question has long existed as to its value in the development of significant bone mineral stores and in the management of osteoporosis. These are really 2 separate questions. In young men and women, bone mineral content develops as a function of growth in body mass and bone loading. There has been extensive study of the effects of various exercise modes upon bone growth and mineral content in the early years of life in men and women, both pre- and postpuberty.[147–155] The effect of both impact loading such as running and of nonimpact exercise such as cycling and swimming appears to clearly favor impact-loading exercise in both young men and women. This advantage appears to hold through early adulthood as measured in elite competitive athletes.[148,156–162] There does seem to be a slight difference between men and women during these later competitive years, with men building slightly more bone than women.[147,148,156,162,163] Even in later years, athletes have greater bone mineral content than nonathletic controls, which demonstrates the value of early life athletic activity, especially for women, who are at greater risk for osteoporosis. The youthful swimmers in most of these studies seem to have higher bone mineral content than nonexercising controls but generally less than athletes practicing gymnastics, cheerleading, or similar activities. The question of the role of aquatic exercise in later years, especially for women at risk for osteoporosis, is more problematic. Bravo and coworkers studied a group of postmenopausal women over a year, with participants performing a specially created aquatic exercise routine emphasizing impact loading, such as jumping and landing in waist-depth water. Though they found a great many positive changes in the study group, including improvements in functional fitness, specifically flexibility, agility, strength/endurance, cardiorespiratory endurance, and gains in psychological well-being, they did not find an increase in either spine or femoral neck bone mineral density as measured through dual-energy x-ray absorptiometry scanning, although femoral neck mineral content did not decrease over the year.[164] A Turkish study did find gains in calcaneal bone density following a 6-month study of aquatic exercise in a group of 41 postmenopausal women but did not study either the spine or femoral neck, both areas of major concern for osteoporotic fractures.[165] A Japanese study of postmenopausal women found that active exercisers preserved better forearm bone mineral density than non-exercisers, with high-impact activity preserving better than low-impact activities such as swimming but again did not study sites of particular concern for fractures.[166] Aquatic exercise does have a fitness role in women at risk for or with osteoporosis because there are considerable data that such programs can build strength and endurance, and there is generally an accompanying improvement in balance skills, self-efficacy, and well-being.[46,47,49,56,164,167–179] Because of the safety of aquatic exercise, the risk of injury during the exercise period is extremely small, and a fall, should it occur, will generally only cause a person to get his or her hair wet. Thus, it is quite reasonable to begin an active exercise regimen in the pool, either through swimming or vertical exercise and, when feasible, transition to a land-based exercise regimen that involves more impact loading.

RELEVANT THERMOREGULATORY EFFECTS AND PREGNANCY

The 2 major compensatory mechanisms that assist cooling in warm air temperatures are peripheral vasodilatation combined with increased cardiac output. These mechanisms work to counterpurposes in warm water, because they facilitate heat gain when the surrounding environment does not allow evaporative and radiant cooling. Immersion at 40°C (104°F), which is a common hot tub temperature, produces a rectal (core) temperature rise that equates to approximately 0.1°F/min of immersion.[180] This is not a problem in the neurologically intact human, because somatic awareness does not promote allowing core temperature rise much beyond 1°C or even less. But when alcohol or other drugs alter awareness, there is a serious risk of hyperthermia in a relatively brief period of time. There is also a risk when the metabolic ability of the tissues to respond is impaired, such as in vascular insufficiency.

Pregnancy creates a special problem, because small rises in core temperature (1.5°C) have been noted to alter the growth of fetal neuronal tissue, although in the study cited, the temperature increases were the result of infectious processes, which may not be entirely relevant to short-term warm water immersion.[181] There have been no reports of fetal abnormalities associated with short, low-level increases in core temperature under 38.9°C.[182] In general, pregnant women are quite sensitive to core temperature elevations and usually depart the hot tub well before core temperature increases are near teratogenic levels.[182] McMurray and coworkers have demonstrated the safe maintenance of core temperature during pregnancy when performing aquatic exercise in 30°C water.[183–186] A prudent guideline might be to limit hot tub immersion in 40°C tubs to periods of less than 15 min for women in whom pregnancy is a consideration. Aquatic exercise at conventional pool temperatures has been shown to be safe during all trimesters of pregnancy and facilitates aerobic conditioning while reducing joint loading.[187] This may be particularly useful in pregnant women with lumbar spine pain. Aquatic exercise at conventional temperatures has also been shown to improve amniotic fluid production, which may be useful.[188]

APPLICATIONS IN PAIN, FIBROMYALGIA, AND PSYCHIATRIC REHABILITATION

Many effects have been observed anecdotally throughout centuries of aquatic environment use for health maintenance and restoration, but they are difficult to study. Predominant among these are the relaxation effect of water immersion and the effect that water immersion has on pain perception. Skin sensory nerve endings are affected, including temperature, touch, and pressure receptors. Sensory overflow has been suggested to be the mechanism by which pain is less well perceived when the affected body part is immersed in water. Pain modulation is consequently affected with a rise in pain threshold, which increases with temperature and water turbulence, producing the known therapeutic effect of agitated whirlpool immersion.

Numerous studies of pain in persons with fibromyalgia have shown statistically significant improvement in pain and function.[168,189–192] A 1998 study of postoperative pain found warm water immersion treatments to reduce pain and possibly promote wound healing.[193]

Studies have shown aquatic exercise to reduce anxiety scores and increase perceived well-being, equal to or superior to the effects noted with land exercise activity.[194,195] Heart rate variability can be analyzed to assess the impact of respiration and autonomic nervous system activity. During relaxation states, heart rate variability demonstrates an autonomic bias toward vagal or parasympathetic nervous system control, whereas during stressed states, the sympathetic nervous system influence predominates. The heart rate variability pattern seen during immersion is that of vagal or parasympathetic control, indicating perhaps an inherent bias toward the relaxation state.[196] In work done in our laboratory studying heart rate variability, peripheral circulation, and core temperature during cool, neutral, and warm water immersion in both young (ages 18 to 30) and older (ages 40 to 65) subjects, we found a dramatic decrease in sympathetic nervous system activity during warm water immersion but less so during neutral immersion and an increase in sympathetic bias during cool water immersion. During warm water immersion we also found a significant increase in sympathovagal balance, the interplay between the 2 components of the autonomic nervous system. Both groups of subjects responded similarly, although the older group had a more muted response. During the same study, we found consistent decreases in diastolic blood pressures and dramatically increased distal circulation.[197]

APPLICATIONS IN OBESITY REHABILITATION

Aquatic exercise would seem to offer the safest and most protective environment for obese individuals due to the buoyancy effects of immersion, which minimizes the risk of joint injury. With body weight reduced to essentially negligible levels, the immersed individual can exercise vigorously and is capable of producing increases in VO_2max in obese individuals over relatively short time periods.[198] Aquatic exercise programs may be highly beneficial in the restoration of fitness in obese patients due to the protective effects against heavy joint loading in the aquatic environment. On dry land, the ability to achieve an aerobic exercise level for sufficient time to produce a conditioning effect may be difficult in this population, and a program that begins in water and moves to land as strength, endurance, and tolerance build may be the most effective method of achieving both conditioning and weight loss. The advantages of aquatic exercise also include the heat-conductive effects of water, which greatly reduce the risk of heat stress when done in cooler pools.[198,199]

CONCLUSION

As research demonstrates, immersing the body in water produces many physiologic effects that have been used therapeutically over centuries of medical history.

Aquatic exercise and rehabilitation remain vastly underused despite their recent increase in popularity. Studies from the Cooper Clinic database of over 30,000 men and women have shown that swimming for exercise produces health and mortality benefits comparable to or even exceeding walking and running.[170,200] These studies assessed the overall health benefits of aquatic exercise with land-based walking and running and found health effects comparable to both land activities, with the potential added value of the broader range of clinical applicability of aquatic activities in specific populations. A review of the Cooper Clinic database of over 40,000 men showed that swimmers had less than half the mortality risk of sedentary men and approximately half the mortality risk of walkers and runners.[200] All of these effects are good reasons to use the aquatic environment in training and rehabilitation.

Aquatic facilities are widely available, and public acceptance is already high, so there are tremendous potential public health benefits to be achieved through programs targeted at the most costly chronic diseases: hypertension, cardiovascular disease, arthritis and other musculoskeletal pathology, obesity, and deconditioning. Aquatic programs for achieving fitness and restoring function may be designed for a broad range of individuals through an understanding of the fundamental principles of aquatic physics and the application of those principles to human physiology. There is truly magic in the water that seems to both preserve and protect health and longevity.

REFERENCES

1. deVierville J. A history of aquatic rehabilitation. In: Cole A, Becker B, eds. *Comprehensive Aquatic Rehabilitation.* 2nd ed. Philadelphia: Butterworth-Heinemann; 2004:1–18.
2. Smith E. Hydrotherapy in arthritis: underwater therapy applied to chronic atrophic arthritis. Paper presented at: 14th Annual Session of the American Congress of Physical Therapy; September 11, 1935; Kansas City, Mo.
3. Lowman CL. *Technique of Underwater Gymnastics: A Study in Practical Application.* Los Angeles: American Publications; 1937.
4. Frontera WR. *DeLisa's Physical Medicine and Rehabilitation: Principles and Practice.* 5th ed. Philadelphia, PA: Lippincott Williams & Wilkins; 2010.
5. Baruch S. *The Principles and Practice of Hydrotherapy. A Guide to the Application of Water in Disease for Students and Practitioners of Medicine.* London: Balliere, Tindall & Cox; 1900.
6. Bloomfield J, Fricker PA, Fitch KD. *Textbook of Science and Medicine in Sport.* Champaign, Ill: Human Kinetics Books; 1992.
7. Harrison RA, Hillman M, Bulstrode S. Loading of the lower limb when walking partially immersed. *Physiotherapy.* 1992;78:164-166.
8. Giancoli D. *Fluids.* 2nd ed. Englewood Cliffs, NJ: Prentice Hall; 1985.
9. Poyhonen T, Keskinen KL, Hautala A, Malkia E. Determination of hydrodynamic drag forces and drag coefficients on human leg/foot model during knee exercise. *Clin Biomech (Bristol, Avon).* 2000;15:256–260.
10. Arborelius M Jr, Balldin UI, Lilja B, Lundgren CE. Hemodynamic changes in man during immersion with the head above water. *Aerosp Med.* 1972;43:592–598.
11. Gabrielsen A, Johansen LB, Norsk P. Central cardiovascular pressures during graded water immersion in humans. *J Appl Physiol.* 1993;75:581–585.
12. Gabrielsen A, Warberg J, Christensen NJ, et al. Arterial pulse pressure and vasopressin release during graded water immersion in humans. *Am J Physiol Regul Integr Comp Physiol.* 2000;278:R1583–1588.
13. Arborelius M Jr, Balldin UI, Lilja B, Lundgren CE. Regional lung function in man during immersion with the head above water. *Aerosp Med.* 1972;43:701–707.
14. Risch WD, Koubenec HJ, Gauer OH, Lange S. Time course of cardiac distension with rapid immersion in a thermo-neutral bath. *Pflugers Arch.* 1978;374:119–120.
15. Schlant RC, Sonneblick EH. Normal physiology of the cardiovascular system. In: Hurst J, ed. *The Heart.* 6th ed. New York: McGraw-Hill; 1986:51.
16. Risch WD, Koubenec HJ, Beckmann U, Lange S, Gauer OH. The effect of graded immersion on heart volume, central venous pressure, pulmonary blood distribution, and heart rate in man. *Pflugers Arch.* 1978;374:115–118.
17. Haffor AS, Mohler JG, Harrison AC. Effects of water immersion on cardiac output of lean and fat male subjects at rest and during exercise. *Aviat Space Environ Med.* 1991;62:123–127.
18. Dressendorfer RH, Morlock JF, Baker DG, Hong SK. Effects of head-out water immersion on cardiorespiratory responses to maximal cycling exercise. *Undersea Biomed Res.* 1976;3:177–187.
19. Weston CF, O'Hare JP, Evans JM, Corrall RJ. Haemodynamic changes in man during immersion in water at different temperatures. *Clin Sci.* 1987;73:613–616.
20. Gleim GW, Nicholas JA. Metabolic costs and heart rate responses to treadmill walking in water at different depths and temperatures. *Am J Sports Med.* 1989;17:248–252.
21. McArdle WD, Katch F, Katch VL. Functional capacity of the cardiovascular system. In: McArdle WD, Katch F, Katch VL, eds. *Exercise Physiology.* 3rd ed. Malvern, PA: Lea & Febiger; 1991:330–331.
22. Tajima F, Sagawa S, Iwamoto J, Miki K, Claybaugh JR, Shiraki K. Renal and endocrine responses in the elderly during head-out water immersion. *Am J Physiol.* 1988;254(pt 2):R977–983.
23. Sheldahl LM, Tristani FE, Clifford PS, Hughes CV, Sobocinski KA, Morris RD. Effect of head-out water immersion on cardiorespiratory response to dynamic exercise. *J Am Coll Cardiol.* 1987;10:1254–1258.
24. Sheldahl LM, Tristani FE, Clifford PS, Kalbfleisch JH, Smits G, Hughes CV. Effect of head-out water immersion on response to exercise training. *J Appl Physiol.* 1986;60:1878–1881.
25. Sheldahl LM, Wann LS, Clifford PS, Tristani FE, Wolf LG, Kalbfleisch JH. Effect of central hypervolemia on cardiac performance during exercise. *J Appl Physiol.* 1984;57:1662–1667.
26. Silvers WM, Rutledge ER, Dolny DG. Peak cardiorespiratory responses during aquatic and land treadmill exercise. *Med Sci Sports Exerc.* 2007;39:969–975.
27. Svedenhag J, Seger J. Running on land and in water: comparative exercise physiology. *Med Sci Sports Exerc.* 1992;24:1155–1160.
28. Coruzzi P, Biggi A, Musiari L, Ravanetti C, Novarini A. Renin-aldosterone system suppression during water immersion in renovascular hypertension. *Clin Sci (Colch).* 1985;68:609–612.
29. Becker BE, Hildenbrand K, Whitcomb RK, Sanders JP. Biophysiologic effects of warm water immersion. *Int J Aquat Res Educ.* 2009;3:24–37.

30. Hildenbrand K, Becker B, Whitcomb R, Sanders J. Age-dependent autonomic changes following immersion in cool, neutral, and warm water temperatures. *Int J Aquat Res Educ.* 2010;4:127–146.

31. Tei C, Tanaka N. Treatment of chronic congestive heart failure to improve their quality of life—clinical study of thermal vasodilation therapy [in Japanese]. *Nihon Naika Gakkai Zasshi.* 1995;84:1475–1482.

32. Cider A, Sunnerhagen KS, Schaufelberger M, Andersson B. Cardiorespiratory effects of warm water immersion in elderly patients with chronic heart failure. *Clin Physiol Funct Imaging.* 2005;25:313–317.

33. Cider A, Svealv BG, Tang MS, Schaufelberger M, Andersson B. Immersion in warm water induces improvement in cardiac function in patients with chronic heart failure. *Eur J Heart Fail.* 2006;8:308–313.

34. Meyer K. Left ventricular dysfunction and chronic heart failure: should aqua therapy and swimming be allowed? *Br J Sports Med.* 2006;40:817–818.

35. Meyer K, Bucking J. Exercise in heart failure: should aqua therapy and swimming be allowed? *Med Sci Sports Exerc.* 2004;36:2017–2023.

36. Meyer K, Leblanc MC. Aquatic therapies in patients with compromised left ventricular function and heart failure. *Clin Invest Med.* 2008;31:E90–97.

37. Mussivand T, Alshaer H, Haddad H, et al. Thermal therapy: a viable adjunct in the treatment of heart failure? *Congest Heart Fail.* 2008;14:180–186.

38. Epstein M. Renal effects of head-out water immersion in humans: a 15-year update. *Physiol Rev.* 1992;72:563–621.

39. Balldin UI, Lundgren CE, Lundvall J, Mellander S. Changes in the elimination of 133 xenon from the anterior tibial muscle in man induced by immersion in water and by shifts in body position. *Aerosp Med.* 1971;42:489–493.

40. Martin WH III, Montgomery J, Snell PG, et al. Cardiovascular adaptations to intense swim training in sedentary middle-aged men and women. *Circulation.* 1987;75:323–330.

41. Ernst E ST, Resch KL. A single blind randomized, controlled trial of hydrotherapy for varicose veins. *Vasa.* 1991;20:147–152.

42. Elmstahl S, Lilja B, Bergqvist D, Brunkwall J. Hydrotherapy of patients with intermittent claudication: a novel approach to improve systolic ankle pressure and reduce symptoms. *Int Angiol.* 1995;14:389–394.

43. Pedersen BK, Saltin B. Evidence for prescribing exercise as therapy in chronic disease. *Scand J Med Sci Sports.* 2006;16(suppl 1):3–63.

44. Silva LE, Valim V, Pessanha AP, et al. Hydrotherapy versus conventional land-based exercise for the management of patients with osteoarthritis of the knee: a randomized clinical trial. *Phys Ther.* 2008;88:12–21.

45. Lund H, Weile U, Christensen R, et al. A randomized controlled trial of aquatic and land-based exercise in patients with knee osteoarthritis. *J Rehabil Med.* 2008;40:137–144.

46. Wang TJ, Belza B, Elaine Thompson F, Whitney JD, Bennett K. Effects of aquatic exercise on flexibility, strength and aerobic fitness in adults with osteoarthritis of the hip or knee. *J Adv Nurs.* 2007;57:141–152.

47. Hinman RS, Heywood SE, Day AR. Aquatic physical therapy for hip and knee osteoarthritis: results of a single-blind randomized controlled trial. *Phys Ther.* 2007;87:32–43.

48. Fransen M, Nairn L, Winstanley J, Lam P, Edmonds J. Physical activity for osteoarthritis management: a randomized controlled clinical trial evaluating hydrotherapy or tai chi classes. *Arthritis Rheum.* 2007;57:407–414.

49. Bartels EM, Lund H, Hagen KB, Dagfinrud H, Christensen R, Danneskiold-Samsoe B. Aquatic exercise for the treatment of knee and hip osteoarthritis. *Cochrane Database Syst Rev.* 2007(4):CD005523.

50. Eversden L, Maggs F, Nightingale P, Jobanputra P. A pragmatic randomised controlled trial of hydrotherapy and land exercises on overall well being and quality of life in rheumatoid arthritis. *BMC Musculoskelet Disord.* 2007;8:23.

51. Verhagen AP, Bierma-Zeinstra SM, Cardoso JR, de Bie RA, Boers M, de Vet HC. Balneotherapy for rheumatoid arthritis. *Cochrane Database Syst Rev.* 2003(4):CD000518.

52. Hall J, Skevington SM, Maddison PJ, Chapman K. A randomized and controlled trial of hydrotherapy in rheumatoid arthritis. *Arthritis Care Res.* 1996;9:206–215.

53. Stenstrom CH. *Dynamic Therapeutic Exercise in Rheumatoid Arthritis* [dissertation]. Stockholm: Rehabilitation and Physical Medicine, Karolinska Institutet; 1993.

54. Bacon MC, Nicholson C, Binder H, White PH. Juvenile rheumatoid arthritis. Aquatic exercise and lower-extremity function. *Arthritis Care Res.* 1991;4:102–105.

55. Minor MA, Hewett JE, Webel RR, Anderson SK, Kay DR. Efficacy of physical conditioning exercise in patients with rheumatoid arthritis and osteoarthritis. *Arthritis Rheum.* 1989;32:1396–1405.

56. Danneskiold-Samsoe B, Lyngberg K, Risum T, Telling M. The effect of water exercise therapy given to patients with rheumatoid arthritis. *Scand J Rehabil Med.* 1987;19:31–35.

57. Frangolias DD, Rhodes EC. Metabolic responses and mechanisms during water immersion running and exercise. *Sports Med.* 1996;22:38–53.

58. Reilly T, Dowzer CN, Cable NT. The physiology of deep-water running. *J Sports Sci.* 2003;21:959–972.

59. Thein JM, Brody LT. Aquatic-based rehabilitation and training for the elite athlete. *J Orthop Sports Phys Ther.* 1998;27:32–41.

60. Wilder RP, Brennan DK. Physiological responses to deep water running in athletes. *Sports Med.* 1993;16:374–380.

61. Haff GG. Aquatic cross training for athletes: part 1. *Strength Cond J.* 2008;30(2):18–26.

62. Becker BE, Lindle-Chewning JM, Huff K, et al. Aquatic cross training for athletes: part 2. *Strength Cond J.* 2008;30(3):67–73.

63. Peyre-Tartaruga LA, Tartaruga MP, Coertjens M, Black GL, Oliveira AR, Kruel LFM. Physiologic and kinematical effects of water run training on running performance. *Int J Aquat Res Educ.* 2009;3:135–150.

64. DeMaere JM, Ruby BC. Effects of deep water and treadmill running on oxygen uptake and energy expenditure in seasonally trained cross country runners. *J Sports Med Phys Fitness.* 1997;37:175–181.

65. Masumoto K, Delion D, Mercer JA. Insight into muscle activity during deep water running. *Med Sci Sports Exerc.* 2009;41(10):1958-1964.

66. Kaneda K, Sato D, Wakabayashi H, Nomura T. EMG activity of hip and trunk muscles during deep-water running. *J Electromyogr Kinesiol.* 2009;19:1064–1070.

67. Kilding AE, Scott MA, Mullineaux DR. A kinematic comparison of deep water running and overground running in endurance runners. *J Strength Cond Res.* 2007;21:476–480.

68. Nakanishi Y, Kimura T, Yokoo Y. Physiological responses to maximal treadmill and deep water running in the young and the middle aged males. *Appl Human Sci.* 1999;18(3):81–86.

69. Gatti CJ, Young RJ, Glad HL. Effect of water-training in the maintenance of cardiorespiratory endurance of athletes. *Br J Sports Med.* 1979;13:161–164.

70. Bushman BA, Flynn MG, Andres FF, Lambert CP, Taylor MS, Braun WA. Effect of 4 wk of deep water run training on running performance. *Med Sci Sports Exerc.* 1997;29:694–699.

71. Wilber RL, Moffatt RJ, Scott BE, Lee DT, Cucuzzo NA. Influence of water run training on the maintenance of aerobic performance. *Med Sci Sports Exerc.* 1996;28:1056–1062.

72. Avellini BA, Shapiro Y, Pandolf KB. Cardio-respiratory physical training in water and on land. *Eur J Appl Physiol Occup Physiol.* 1983;50:255–263.

73. Killgore GL, Wilcox AR, Caster BL, Wood TM. A lower-extremities kinematic comparison of deep-water running styles and treadmill running. *J Strength Cond Res.* 2006;20:919–927.

74. Robinson LE, Devor ST, Merrick MA, Buckworth J. The effects of land vs. aquatic plyometrics on power, torque, velocity, and muscle soreness in women. *J Strength Cond Res.* 2004;18:84–91.

75. Martel GF, Harmer ML, Logan JM, Parker CB. Aquatic plyometric training increases vertical jump in female volleyball players. *Med Sci Sports Exerc.* 2005;37:1814–1819.

76. Pantoja PD, Alberton CL, Pilla C, Vendrusculo AP, Kruel LF. Effect of resistive exercise on muscle damage in water and on land. *J Strength Cond Res.* 2009;23:1051–1054.

77. Dundar U, Solak O, Yigit I, Evcik D, Kavuncu V. Clinical effectiveness of aquatic exercise to treat chronic low back pain: a randomized controlled trial. *Spine (Phila Pa 1976).* 2009;34:1436–1440.

78. Olah M, Molnar L, Dobai J, Olah C, Feher J, Bender T. The effects of weightbath traction hydrotherapy as a component of complex physical therapy in disorders of the cervical and lumbar spine: a controlled pilot study with follow-up. *Rheumatol Int.* 2008;28:749–756.

79. Cole A, Frederickson M, Johnson J, Moschetti M, Eagleston R, Stratton S. Spine pain: aquatic rehabilitation strategies. In: Cole C, Becker B, eds. *Comprehensive Aquatic Therapy.* 2nd ed. Philadelphia: Butterworth Heinemann; 2004:177–206.

80. Guillemin F, Constant F, Collin JF, Boulange M. Short and long-term effect of spa therapy in chronic low back pain. *Br J Rheumatol.* 1994;33:148–151.

81. Becker B. Aquatic therapy in the management of spinal disorders. *Spine Line.* March/April 2002;19–22.

82. Waller B, Lambeck J, Daly D. Therapeutic aquatic exercise in the treatment of low back pain: a systematic review. *Clin Rehabil.* 2009;23:3–14.

83. Hong SK, Cerretelli P, Cruz JC, Rahn H. Mechanics of respiration during submersion in water. *J Appl Physiol.* 1969;27:535–538.

84. Agostoni E, Gurtner G, Torri G, Rahn H. Respiratory mechanics during submersion and negative-pressure breathing. *J Appl Physiol.* 1966;21:251–258.

85. Taylor NA, Morrison JB. Pulmonary flow-resistive work during hydrostatic loading. *Acta Physiol Scand.* 1991;142:307–312.

86. Taylor NA, Morrison JB. Static and dynamic pulmonary compliance during upright immersion. *Acta Physiol Scand.* 1993;149:413–417.

87. Taylor NA, Morrison JB. Static respiratory muscle work during immersion with positive and negative respiratory loading. *J Appl Physiol.* 1999;87:1397–1403.

88. Mangelsdorff G, Borzone G, Leiva A, Martinez A, Lisboa C. Strength of inspiratory muscles in chronic heart failure and chronic pulmonary obstructive disease [in Spanish]. *Rev Med Chil.* 2001;129:51–59.

89. Dempsey JA, Miller JD, Romer L, Amann M, Smith CA. Exercise-induced respiratory muscle work: effects on blood flow, fatigue and performance. *Adv Exp Med Biol.* 2008;605:209–212.

90. Dempsey JA, Amann M, Romer LM, Miller JD. Respiratory system determinants of peripheral fatigue and endurance performance. *Med Sci Sports Exerc.* 2008;40:457–461.

91. Dempsey JA, Romer L, Rodman J, Miller J, Smith C. Consequences of exercise-induced respiratory muscle work. *Respir Physiol Neurobiol.* 28 2006;151:242–250.

92. McConnell AK, Romer LM. Respiratory muscle training in healthy humans: resolving the controversy. *Int J Sports Med.* 2004;25:284–293.

93. Litchke LG, Russian CJ, Lloyd LK, Schmidt EA, Price L, Walker JL. Effects of respiratory resistance training with a concurrent flow device on wheelchair athletes. *J Spinal Cord Med.* 2008;31:65–71.

94. Witt JD, Guenette JA, Rupert JL, McKenzie DC, Sheel AW. Inspiratory muscle training attenuates the human respiratory muscle metaboreflex. *J Physiol.* 2007;584(pt 3):1019–1028.

95. Lindholm P, Wylegala J, Pendergast DR, Lundgren CE. Resistive respiratory muscle training improves and maintains endurance swimming performance in divers. *Undersea Hyperb Med.* 2007;34(3):169–180.

96. Johnson MA, Sharpe GR, Brown PI. Inspiratory muscle training improves cycling time-trial performance and anaerobic work capacity but not critical power. *Eur J Appl Physiol.* 2007;101:761–770.

97. Griffiths LA, McConnell AK. The influence of inspiratory and expiratory muscle training upon rowing performance. *Eur J Appl Physiol.* 2007;99:457–466.

98. Padula CA, Yeaw E. Inspiratory muscle training: integrative review. *Res Theory Nurs Pract.* 2006;20:291–304.

99. Guenette JA, Martens AM, Lee AL, et al. Variable effects of respiratory muscle training on cycle exercise performance in men and women. *Appl Physiol Nutr Metab.* 2006;31:159–166.

100. Enright SJ, Unnithan VB, Heward C, Withnall L, Davies DH. Effect of high-intensity inspiratory muscle training on lung volumes, diaphragm thickness, and exercise capacity in subjects who are healthy. *Phys Ther.* 2006;86:345–354.

101. McConnell AK, Sharpe GR. The effect of inspiratory muscle training upon maximum lactate steady-state and blood lactate concentration. *Eur J Appl Physiol.* 2005;94:277–284.

102. Gething AD, Williams M, Davies B. Inspiratory resistive loading improves cycling capacity: a placebo controlled trial. *Br J Sports Med.* 2004;38:730–736.

103. Gething AD, Passfield L, Davies B. The effects of different inspiratory muscle training intensities on exercising heart rate and perceived exertion. *Eur J Appl Physiol.* 2004;92:50–55.

104. Romer LM, McConnell AK, Jones DA. Effects of inspiratory muscle training on time-trial performance in trained cyclists. *J Sports Sci.* 2002;20:547–562.

105. Romer LM, McConnell AK, Jones DA. Inspiratory muscle fatigue in trained cyclists: effects of inspiratory muscle training. *Med Sci Sports Exerc.* 2002;34:785–792.

106. Romer LM, McConnell AK, Jones DA. Effects of inspiratory muscle training upon recovery time during high intensity, repetitive sprint activity. *Int J Sports Med.* 2002;23:353–360.

107. Volianitis S, McConnell AK, Koutedakis Y, McNaughton L, Backx K, Jones DA. Inspiratory muscle training improves rowing performance. *Med Sci Sports Exerc.* 2001;33:803–809.

108. Sonetti DA, Wetter TJ, Pegelow DF, Dempsey JA. Effects of respiratory muscle training versus placebo on endurance exercise performance. *Respir Physiol.* 2001;127:185–199.

109. Inbar O, Weiner P, Azgad Y, Rotstein A, Weinstein Y. Specific inspiratory muscle training in well-trained endurance athletes. *Med Sci Sports Exerc.* 2000;32:1233–1237.

110. Volianitis S, McConnell AK, Koutedakis Y, Jones DA. Specific respiratory warm-up improves rowing performance and exertional dyspnea. *Med Sci Sports Exerc.* 2001;33:1189–1193.

111. Clanton TL, Dixon GF, Drake J, Gadek JE. Effects of swim training on lung volumes and inspiratory muscle conditioning. *J Appl Physiol.* 1987;62:39–46.

112. Mickleborough TD, Stager JM, Chatham K, Lindley MR, Ionescu AA. Pulmonary adaptations to swim and inspiratory muscle training. *Eur J Appl Physiol.* 2008;103:635–646.

113. Wells GD, Plyley M, Thomas S, Goodman L, Duffin J. Effects of concurrent inspiratory and expiratory muscle training on respiratory and exercise performance in competitive swimmers. *Eur J Appl Physiol.* 2005;94:527–540.

114. Bjurstrom RL, Schoene RB. Control of ventilation in elite synchronized swimmers. *J Appl Physiol.* 1987;63:1019–1024.

115. Cordain L, Tucker A, Moon D, Stager JM. Lung volumes and maximal respiratory pressures in collegiate swimmers and runners. *Res Q Exerc Sport.* 1990;61:70–74.

116. Courteix D, Obert P, Lecoq AM, Guenon P, Koch G. Effect of intensive swimming training on lung volumes, airway resistance and on the maximal expiratory flow-volume relationship in prepubertal girls. *Eur J Appl Physiol Occup Physiol.* 1997;76:264–269.

117. Engstrom I, Eriksson BO, Karlberg P, Saltin B, Thoren C. Preliminary report on the development of lung volumes in young girl swimmers. *Acta Paediatr Scand Suppl.* 1971;217:73–76.

118. Hill NS, Jacoby C, Farber HW. Effect of an endurance triathlon on pulmonary function. *Med Sci Sports Exerc.* 1991;23:1260–1264.

119. Kesavachandran C, Nair HR, Shashidhar S. Lung volumes in swimmers performing different styles of swimming. *Indian J Med Sci.* 2001;55:669–676.

120. Cordain L, Stager J. Pulmonary structure and function in swimmers. *Sports Med.* 1988;6:271–278.

121. Doherty M, Dimitriou L. Comparison of lung volume in Greek swimmers, land based athletes, and sedentary controls using allometric scaling. *Br J Sports Med.* 1997;31:337–341.

122. Magel JR. Comparison of the physiologic response to varying intensities of submaximal work in tethered swimming and treadmill running. *J Sports Med Phys Fitness.* 1971;11:203–212.

123. Zinman R, Gaultier C. Maximal static pressures and lung volumes in young female swimmers. *Respir Physiol.* 1986;64:229–239.

124. Zinman R, Gaultier C. Maximal static pressures and lung volumes in young female swimmers: one year follow-up. *Pediatr Pulmonol.* 1987;3(3):145–148.

125. Dempsey JA, Sheel AW, St Croix CM, Morgan BJ. Respiratory influences on sympathetic vasomotor outflow in humans. *Respir Physiol Neurobiol.* 2002;130:3–20.

126. Sheel AW, Derchak PA, Morgan BJ, Pegelow DF, Jacques AJ, Dempsey JA. Fatiguing inspiratory muscle work causes reflex reduction in resting leg blood flow in humans. *J Physiol.* 2001;537(pt 1):277–289.

127. Sheel AW, Derchak PA, Pegelow DF, Dempsey JA. Threshold effects of respiratory muscle work on limb vascular resistance. *Am J Physiol.* 2002;282:H1732–1738.

128. Miller JD, Smith CA, Hemauer SJ, Dempsey JA. The effects of inspiratory intrathoracic pressure production on the cardiovascular response to submaximal exercise in health and chronic heart failure. *Am J Physiol.* 2007;292:H580–592.

129. Watsford ML, Murphy AJ, Pine MJ, Coutts AJ. The effect of habitual exercise on respiratory-muscle function in older adults. *J Aging Phys Act.* 2005;13:34–44.

130. McConnell AK, Weiner P, Romer LM. Inspiratory muscle training as a tool for the management of patients with COPD. *Eur Respir J.* 2004;24:510–511; author reply 511.

131. McConnell AK, Romer LM. Dyspnoea in health and obstructive pulmonary disease: the role of respiratory muscle function and training. *Sports Med.* 2004;34:117–132.

132. Covey MK, Larson JL, Wirtz SE, et al. High-intensity inspiratory muscle training in patients with chronic obstructive pulmonary disease and severely reduced function. *J Cardiopulm Rehabil.* 2001;21:231–240.

133. Liaw MY, Lin MC, Cheng PT, Wong MK, Tang FT. Resistive inspiratory muscle training: its effectiveness in patients with acute complete cervical cord injury. *Arch Phys Med Rehabil.* 2000;81:752–756.

134. O'Brien K, Geddes EL, Reid WD, Brooks D, Crowe J. Inspiratory muscle training compared with other rehabilitation interventions in chronic obstructive pulmonary disease: a systematic review update. *J Cardiopulm Rehabil Prev.* 2008;28:128–141.

135. Garcia S, Rocha M, Pinto P, Lopes AMF, Barbara C. Inspiratory muscle training in COPD patients. *Rev Port Pneumol.* 2008;14:177–194.

136. Magadle R, McConnell AK, Beckerman M, Weiner P. Inspiratory muscle training in pulmonary rehabilitation program in COPD patients. *Respir Med.* 2007;101:1500–1505.

137. Crisafulli E, Costi S, Fabbri LM, Clini EM. Respiratory muscles training in COPD patients. *Int J Chron Obstruct Pulmon Dis.* 2007;2:19–25.

138. Hill K, Jenkins SC, Philippe DL, et al. High-intensity inspiratory muscle training in COPD. *Eur Respir J.* 2006;27:1119–1128.

139. Adams MA, Chandler LS. Effects of physical therapy program on vital capacity of patients with muscular dystrophy. *Phys Ther.* 1974;54:494–496.

140. Koessler W, Wanke T, Winkler G, et al. 2 Years' experience with inspiratory muscle training in patients with neuromuscular disorders. *Chest.* 2001;120:765–769.

141. Topin N, Matecki S, Le Bris S, et al. Dose-dependent effect of individualized respiratory muscle training in children with Duchenne muscular dystrophy. *Neuromuscul Disord.* 2002;12:576–583.

142. Wanke T, Toifl K, Merkle M, Formanek D, Lahrmann H, Zwick H. Inspiratory muscle training in patients with Duchenne muscular dystrophy. *Chest.* 1994;105:475–482.

143. Pachalski A, Mekarski T. Effect of swimming on increasing of cardio-respiratory capacity in paraplegics. *Paraplegia.* 1980;18:190–196.

144. Van Houtte S, Vanlandewijck Y, Gosselink R. Respiratory muscle training in persons with spinal cord injury: a systematic review. *Respir Med.* 2006;100:1886–1895.

145. Kaneda K, Sato D, Wakabayashi H, Hanai A, Nomura T. A Comparison of the effects of different water exercise programs on balance ability in elderly people. *J Aging Phys Act.* 2008;16:381–392.

146. Suomi R, Koceja DM. Postural sway characteristics in women with lower extremity arthritis before and after an aquatic exercise intervention. *Arch Phys Med Rehabil.* 2000;81:780–785.

147. Tsuji S, Akama H. Weight training may provide a better stimulus for increasing bone mineral content (BMC) than run and swimming training. *Med Science Sports Exerc.* 1991;23:882–883.

148. Orwoll ES, Ferar J, Oviatt SK, McClung MR, Huntington K. The relationship of swimming exercise to bone mass in men and women. *Arch Intern Med.* 1989;149:2197–2200.

149. Hara S, Yanagi H, Amagai H, Endoh K, Tsuchiya S, Tomura S. Effect of physical activity during teenage years, based on type of sport and duration of exercise, on bone mineral density of young, premenopausal Japanese women. *Calcif Tissue Int.* 2001;68:23–30.

150. Falk B, Bronshtein Z, Zigel L, Constantini NW, Eliakim A. Quantitative ultrasound of the tibia and radius in prepubertal and early-pubertal female athletes. *Arch Pediatr Adolesc Med.* 2003;157:139–143.

151. Falk B, Bronshtein Z, Zigel L, Constantini N, Eliakim A. Higher tibial quantitative ultrasound in young female swimmers. *Br J Sports Med.* 2004;38:461–465.

152. Duncan CS, Blimkie CJ, Cowell CT, Burke ST, Briody JN, Howman-Giles R. Bone mineral density in adolescent female athletes: relationship to exercise type and muscle strength. *Med Sci Sports Exerc.* 2002;34:286–294.

153. Derman O, Cinemre A, Kanbur N, Dogan M, Kilic M, Karaduman E. Effect of swimming on bone metabolism in adolescents. *Turk J Pediatr.* 2008;50:149–154.

154. Chu KS, Rhodes EC. Physiological and cardiovascular changes associated with deep water running in the young. Possible implications for the elderly. *Sports Med.* 2001;31:33–46.

155. Bellew JW, Gehrig L. A comparison of bone mineral density in adolescent female swimmers, soccer players, and weight lifters. *Pediatr Phys Ther.* 2006;18:19–22.

156. Taaffe DR, Marcus R. Regional and total body bone mineral density in elite collegiate male swimmers. *J Sports Med Phys Fitness.* 1999;39:154–159.

157. Heinrich CH, Going SB, Pamenter RW, Perry CD, Boyden TW, Lohman TG. Bone mineral content of cyclically menstruating female resistance and endurance trained athletes. *Med Sci Sports Exerc.* 1990;22:558–563.

158. Fehling PC, Alekel L, Clasey J, Rector A, Stillman RJ. A comparison of bone mineral densities among female athletes in impact loading and active loading sports. *Bone.* 1995;17:205–210.

159. Emslander HC, Sinaki M, Muhs JM, et al. Bone mass and muscle strength in female college athletes (runners and swimmers). *Mayo Clin Proc.* 1998;73:1151–1160.

160. Dook JE, James C, Henderson NK, Price RI. Exercise and bone mineral density in mature female athletes. *Med Sci Sports Exerc.* 1997;29:291–296.

161. Creighton DL, Morgan AL, Boardley D, Brolinson PG. Weight-bearing exercise and markers of bone turnover in female athletes. *J Appl Physiol.* 2001;90:565–570.

162. Avlonitou E, Georgiou E, Douskas G, Louizi A. Estimation of body composition in competitive swimmers by means of three different techniques. *Int J Sports Med.* 1997;18:363–368.

163. Magkos F, Kavouras SA, Yannakoulia M, Karipidou M, Sidossi S, Sidossis LS. The bone response to non-weight-bearing exercise is sport-, site-, and sex-specific. *Clin J Sport Med.* 2007;17:123–128.

164. Bravo G, Gauthier P, Roy PM, Payette H, Gaulin P. A weight-bearing, water-based exercise program for osteopenic women: its impact on bone, functional fitness, and well-being. *Arch Phys Med Rehabil.* 1997;78:1375–1380.

165. Ay A, Yurtkuran M. Evaluation of hormonal response and ultrasonic changes in the heel bone by aquatic exercise in sedentary postmenopausal women. *Am J Phys Med Rehabil.* 2003;82:942–949.

166. Nagata M, Kitagawa J, Miyake T, Nakahara Y. Effects of exercise practice on the maintenance of radius bone mineral density in postmenopausal women. *J Physiol Anthropol Appl Human Sci.* 2002;21:229–234.

167. Ariyoshi M, Sonoda K, Nagata K, et al. Efficacy of aquatic exercises for patients with low-back pain. *Kurume Med J.* 1999;46:91–96.

168. Assis MR, Silva LE, Alves AM, et al. A randomized controlled trial of deep water running: clinical effectiveness of aquatic exercise to treat fibromyalgia. *Arthritis Rheum.* 2006;55:57–65.

169. Barbosa TM, Garrido MF, Bragada J. Physiological adaptations to head-out aquatic exercises with different levels of body immersion. *J Strength Cond Res.* 2007;21:1255–1259.

170. Chase NL, Sui X, Blair SN. Comparison of the health aspects of swimming with other types of physical activity and sedentary lifestyle habits. *Int J Aquat Res Educ.* 2008;2:151–161.

171. Gehlsen GM, Grigsby SA, Winant DM. Effects of an aquatic fitness program on the muscular strength and endurance of patients with multiple sclerosis. *Phys Ther.* 1984;64:653–657.

172. Gusi N, Tomas-Carus P, Hakkinen A, Hakkinen K, Ortega-Alonso A. Exercise in waist-high warm water decreases pain and improves health-related quality of life and strength in the lower extremities in women with fibromyalgia. *Arthritis Rheum.* 2006;55:66–73.

173. Jentoft ES, Kvalvik AG, Mengshoel AM. Effects of pool-based and land-based aerobic exercise on women with fibromyalgia/chronic widespread muscle pain. *Arthritis Rheum.* 2001;45:42–47.

174. Lin SY, Davey RC, Cochrane T. Community rehabilitation for older adults with osteoarthritis of the lower limb: a controlled clinical trial. *Clin Rehabil.* 2004;18:92–101.

175. Seynnes O, Hue O, Ledrole D, Bernard PL. Adapted physical activity in old age: effects of a low-intensity training program on isokinetic power and fatigability. *Aging Clin Exp Res.* 2002;14:491–498.

176. Stenstrom CH, Lindell B, Swanberg E, Swanberg P, Harms-Ringdahl K, Nordemar R. Intensive dynamic training in water for rheumatoid arthritis functional class II—a long-term study of effects. *Scand J Rheumatol.* 1991;20:358–365.

177. Suomi R, Collier D. Effects of arthritis exercise programs on functional fitness and perceived activities of daily living measures in older adults with arthritis. *Arch Phys Med Rehabil.* 2003;84:1589–1594.

178. Templeton MS, Booth DL, O'Kelly WD. Effects of aquatic therapy on joint flexibility and functional ability in subjects with rheumatic disease. *J Orthop Sports Phys Ther.* 1996;23:376–381.

179. Tsourlou T, Benik A, Dipla K, Zafeiridis A, Kellis S. The effects of a twenty-four-week aquatic training program on muscular strength performance in healthy elderly women. *J Strength Cond Res.* 2006;20:811–818.

180. Allison TG, Reger WE. Comparison of responses of men to immersion in circulating water at 40.0 and 41.5 degrees C. *Aviat Space Environ Med.* 1998;69:845–850.

181. Smith DW, Clarren SK, Harvey MA. Hyperthermia as a possible teratogenic agent. *J Pediatr.* 1978;92:878–883.

182. Harvey MA, McRorie MM, Smith DW. Suggested limits to the use of the hot tub and sauna by pregnant women. *Can Med Assoc J.* 1981;125:50–53.

183. McMurray RG, Berry MJ, Katz VL, Graetzer DG, Cefalo RC. The thermoregulation of pregnant women during aerobic exercise in the water: a longitudinal approach. *Eur J Appl Physiol Occup Physiol.* 1990;61:119–123.

184. McMurray RG, Katz VL. Thermoregulation in pregnancy. Implications for exercise. *Sports Med.* 1990;10:146–158.

185. McMurray RG, Katz VL, Berry MJ, Cefalo RC. Cardiovascular responses of pregnant women during aerobic exercise in water: a longitudinal study. *Int J Sports Med.* 1988;9:443–447.

186. McMurray RG, Katz VL, Meyer-Goodwin WE, Cefalo RC. Thermoregulation of pregnant women during aerobic exercise on land and in the water. *Am J Perinatol.* 1993;10:178–182.

187. Hartmann S, Bung P. Physical exercise during pregnancy—physiological considerations and recommendations. *J Perinat Med.* 1999;27:204–215.

188. San Juan Dertkigil M, Cecatti JG, Sarno MA, Cavalcante SR, Marussi EF. Variation in the amniotic fluid index following moderate physical activity in water during pregnancy. *Acta Obstet Gynecol Scand.* 2007;86:547–552.

189. Busch A, Schachter CL, Peloso PM, Bombardier C. Exercise for treating fibromyalgia syndrome. *Cochrane Database Syst Rev.* 2002(3):CD003786.

190. Gowans SE, deHueck A. Pool exercise for individuals with fibromyalgia. *Curr Opin Rheumatol.* 2007;19:168–173.

191. McCain GA. Nonmedicinal treatments in primary fibromyalgia. *Rheum Dis Clin North Am.* 1989;15:73–90.

192. Tomas-Carus P, Hakkinen A, Gusi N, Leal A, Hakkinen K, Ortega-Alonso A. Aquatic training and detraining on fitness and quality of life in fibromyalgia. *Med Sci Sports Exerc.* 2007;39:1044–1050.

193. Juve Meeker B. Whirlpool therapy on postoperative pain and surgical wound healing: an exploration. *Patient Educ Couns.* 1998;33:39–48.

194. Robiner WN. Psychological and physical reactions to whirlpool baths. *J Behav Med.* 1990;13:157–173.

195. Watanabe E, Takeshima N, Okada A, Inomata K. Comparison of water- and land-based exercise in the reduction of state anxiety among older adults. *Percept Mot Skills.* 2000;91:97–104.

196. Perini R, Milesi S, Biancardi L, Pendergast DR, Veicsteinas A. Heart rate variability in exercising humans: effect of water immersion. *Eur J Appl Physiol.* 1998;77:326–332.

197. Becker B, Hildenbrand K, Whitcomb B, Sanders J. Biophysiologic effects of warm water immersion. *Int J Aquat Res Educ.* 2009;3:24-37.

198. Sheldahl LM. Special ergometric techniques and weight reduction. *Med Sci Sports Exerc.* 1986;18:25–30.

199. Xu X, Castellani JW, Santee W, Kolka M. Thermal responses for men with different fat compositions during immersion in cold water at two depths: prediction versus observation. *Eur J Appl Physiol.* 2007;100:79–88.

200. Chase NL, Sui X, Blair SN. Swimming and all-cause mortality risk compared with running, walking and sedentary habits in men. *Int J Aquat Res Educ.* 2008;2:213–223.

2

Guidelines and Indications for the Use of Aquatic Therapy

Jessica Heath, PT, OCS, Cert MDT, CSCS and Lisa Pataky, PT, DPT

Water is an excellent medium for achieving maximal exercise levels in those with or without disabilities. As previously mentioned, water has several unique qualities, such as buoyancy, hydrostatic pressure, thermodynamics, and specific gravity, that make aquatic therapy an ideal choice for individuals with musculoskeletal, cardiopulmonary, or neurological impairments as well as individuals with general deconditioning and debility. Aquatic therapy can be used for both acute and chronic conditions.[1] Aquatic therapy provides a useful and safe environment for initiating an exercise therapy program and can complement all phases of the rehabilitation process while providing a margin of therapeutic safety that is wider than almost any other type of treatment environment.[1] The physical properties of water provide certain benefits to patients that land-based programs do not offer, making aquatic therapy the ideal rehabilitation environment for many individuals and conditions.

Aquatic therapy uses the physical properties of water to provide assistive, supportive, or resistive exercises.[2,3] Assistive exercises occur when movements are toward the surface of the water and can be used when wanting to increase range of motion (ROM) and flexibility of joints.[3] Supportive exercises involve those that occur in a direction perpendicular to the upward thrust of buoyancy or parallel to the bottom of the pool.[3] Examples of this type of exercise include glenohumeral horizontal abduction/adduction while standing or hip abduction/adduction in supine. Resistive exercises occur by opposing the force of buoyancy by moving a body part away from the surface of the water.[3] Hip extension in standing beginning at 90 degrees of

flexion and extending to neutral is an example of a resistive strengthening exercise (Figure 2-1).

The properties of viscosity and fluid resistance allow the resistance of exercises to easily be altered by merely changing the position of a limb, speed of movement, or direction of movement.[3] Any change in limb speed or direction therefore changes the resistance felt, and because human motion is highly variable in its direction and velocity, greater functional gains can be made from resistance exercises via aquatic therapy.[4] Aquatic strengthening exercises can be designed in a way that closely mimics everyday movements to allow for neuromuscular adaptations that can help decrease levels of difficulty with completing activities of daily living (ADL).[4] Water also has accommodating resistance, meaning that the resistance of the water is matched to the individual's applied force or effort.[4] Therefore, the likelihood of exacerbation of symptoms or reinjury is significantly decreased, as most individuals will not exert enough force to reach those levels.

The property of specific gravity aids in the flotation of individuals once in the water, with individuals with lower specific gravity (those with a greater percentage of adipose tissue) floating more easily and those with higher specific gravity (those with a high percentage of lean body tissue) floating less easily and possibly requiring flotation devices for assistance.[1,3] The thermal conductive properties of water increase the versatility of aquatic therapy because different goals can be achieved using colder or warmer water temperatures. Water retains heat or cold while delivering it easily to the immersed body part; therefore, therapy in colder water temperatures can be used to decrease muscle pain and speed recovery from overuse injuries,[1] whereas

Wilk KE, Joyner DM. *The Use of Aquatics in Orthopedic and Sports Medicine Rehabilitation and Physical Conditioning (pp 17-26).*
© 2014 SLACK Incorporated.

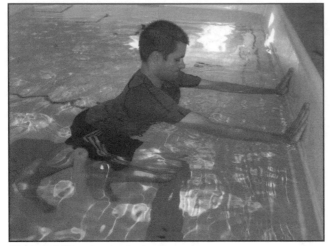

Figure 2-1. Hip extension in standing.

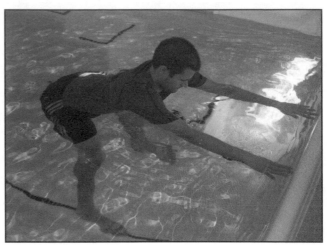

Figure 2-2. Squat against wall.

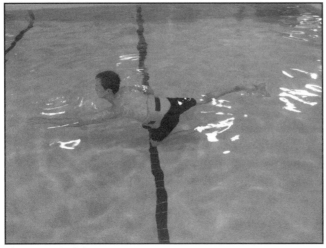

Figure 2-3. Bird dog.

warmer water therapy can be used for muscle relaxation, increased blood flow to muscles and tissues, and decreased feelings of pain and discomfort.[1,5]

Typical therapy pools are kept between 33.5°C and 35.5°C (92.3°F and 96°F), allowing for extended immersion time to provide optimal therapeutic benefits without the risk of overheating or cooling.[1] One of the main benefits of the use of water in therapy is that it decreases the gravitational forces placed on joints, allowing for decreased joint stresses and weight bearing. When an individual is submerged to the level of the anterior–superior iliac spine, he or she is bearing approximately 50% of his or her weight, at the level of the xyphoid process he or she is bearing approximately 30% of his or her weight, and at the level of the clavicle he or she is only experiencing about 10% of his or her body weight.[3]

The buoyancy of water can assist in improving both active and passive ROM while providing an environment in which axial and compressive forces are reduced, thus allowing for earlier initiation of a rehabilitation program.[4] Aquatic therapy also encourages increased motion of the affected limb because the majority of motions that take place in water involve alternating or symmetrical limb movement, which requires the involved side to match the effort and ROM of the uninvolved one.[4] When designing an aquatic therapy program, the impairment, pathology (if known), age of the individual, body composition, and patient's comfort level in the water should all be taken into consideration.

INDICATIONS FOR USE IN ORTHOPEDIC POPULATIONS

Aquatic therapy is very useful for individuals with orthopedic injuries because it can help facilitate earlier return to function with less pain than would be achieved using only traditional, land-based therapy. Individuals who are immobilized after an injury or surgery are predisposed to muscle atrophy, aerobic deconditioning, soft tissue weakness, and decreased joint mobility.[5] Many of these impairments can be offset by early initiation of physical therapy; however, this is not always possible secondary to limitations in ROM, active muscle contraction, or weight bearing. Aquatic therapy provides an excellent way of initiating early rehabilitation in these individuals, and early function-based therapy has been shown to be superior for returning to prior level of function than early immobilization.[5] Aquatic therapy is often indicated when weight-bearing activities are limited or restricted as both closed and open kinetic chain activities can be initiated early on in the water.[5] Shallow water exercises, such as squats (Figure 2-2) and lunges, more closely resemble closed kinetic chain exercises but with reduced joint loading, whereas deep water and horizontal exercises (Figure 2-3) better simulate open kinetic chain activities.[1]

Aquatic therapy provides several benefits such as decreased pain, joint loading, and swelling; improved ROM, endurance, and strength via early initiation of movement; as well as the maintenance or improvement in cardiovascular and aerobic fitness.[1,3–10]

Several theories have been offered to explain how exercise therapy in water helps to decrease feelings of pain and discomfort. Becker suggested that individuals have improved control over their ability to perform exercises within a pain-free range because the force of water drops immediately upon discontinuation of a movement.[1] Therefore, if a patient is experiencing pain, he or she can merely stop the activity to experience a sudden and exponential decrease in pain level, which is not always the case with land-based exercises.[1] Another explanation is that with water immersion, the perception of pain may be dampened due to the sensory overflow that is experienced while in water. Decreased perception of pain can lead to pain modulation and eventually to increased pain thresholds.[1] This sensory overflow and subsequent pain modulation are increased with increased water temperatures and water turbulence.[1] Patients with very high levels of pain or low pain thresholds may benefit most from warmer temperatures with higher water turbulence such as whirlpools. Additionally, the warmth of the water may reduce pain by increasing blood flow to the submerged body parts, allowing for muscle relaxation, and hydrostatic pressure can help to decrease swelling and dampen sympathetic nervous system activity, thus decreasing the feelings of pain.[5]

Decreased swelling and joint loading can also contribute to decreased feelings of pain. The hydrostatic pressure of water is the main force that assists in decreasing swelling when an individual is in water.[1,3] The increased pressure on the thorax and chest cavity results in a shift in blood volume cranially from the lower extremities and abdomen. This superior shift results in central hypervolemia and viscosity, which promote venous return and decreased swelling.[8] As a body is further immersed, more water is displaced, creating an increased force of buoyancy.[1] This increased buoyancy serves to off-load the joints and allows for the performance of functional closed-chain (weight bearing) activities that otherwise might not be possible on land.[1,6] Additionally, because a greater percentage of the body is immersed in water, the individual feels a smaller percentage of their body weight.[1]

Early initiation of movement is critical to the successful rehabilitation of most orthopedic injuries including both those who require surgery and those who do not. Active ROM exercises, gait, and strengthening often may not be initiated until a month or more into traditional, land-based therapy secondary to postoperative restrictions in weight bearing or active muscle contraction. Aquatic therapy offers the benefit of earlier initiation of movement because gravitational forces can be partially or completely offset by the buoyancy effects of water.[1] The only force acting on the joints then would be muscle torque forces, which could allow for earlier initiation of active-assisted ROM, gentle strengthening, and gait training.[1] This ability to initiate these activities earlier can lead to increased improvements in strength and endurance as well as an earlier return to normal gait mechanics, all of which are essential to a return to prior levels of function.

Aquatic therapy offers several cardiovascular and aerobic benefits as well. After only 3 weeks of inactivity, cardiovascular deficits begin, and 6 weeks of rest can lead to a 14% to 16% decrease in maximum oxygen uptake.[3] The opportunity that aquatic therapy provides to return to exercise sooner allows for the maintenance of or improvement in an individual's preinjury fitness level. Warm water allows for increased blood flow and delivery of oxygen to muscles,[7] allowing for improved ability to exercise in aquatic environments. Oxygen availability can increase as much as 22.5% compared to exercising on land.[1] Additionally, studies show that exercising in aquatic environments results in decreased max heart rate and oxygen consumption (VO_2) for the same levels of intensity,[8] meaning that individuals can exercise at higher intensity levels while still maintaining a safe exercise environment.

Aquatic therapy achieves all of these benefits while providing a safe environment that minimizes risk of falls and reinjury.[1] Aquatic therapy can be used as an adjunct or precursor to land-based therapy rather than as a replacement for it. Aquatic therapy allows individuals to begin certain aspects of rehabilitation sooner, and studies show that though there is no difference in the total amount of improvements in individuals participating in land-based versus aquatic therapy, those who participated in aquatic therapy experienced improvements more rapidly.[5] Participants in aquatic therapy can perform better and experience less pain than with traditional land-based therapy due in part to the decreased joint forces and weight bearing that the properties of water allow.[5] Gait mechanics can also be simulated during hydrotherapy without the associated risks of gravitational forces or loss of balance.[4] Though an individual may be under weight-bearing restrictions due to the nature of the injury and therefore unable to ambulate without an assistive device on land, he or she can initiate an aquatic walking program and begin to return to normal, independent walking.

Initiation of rehabilitation via aquatic therapy with later transition to traditional land-based therapy is often indicated when strengthening of a joint or surrounding muscle groups would place too much axial and compressive forces on the injured joints, such as when recovering from back, hip, knee, or ankle injuries.[4] Strengthening can proceed at a more gradual pace in the water and can provide an excellent environment in which to initiate early gentle strengthening exercises without fear of further injury to the involved structures. Aquatic therapy as a precursor to land-based therapy is also indicated if land-based therapy exercises exacerbate the patient's symptoms too much and ROM and gentle strengthening exercises are indicated but not possible with traditional physical therapy.[4] For acute injuries such as stress fractures, strains, and sprains, an individual would want to exercise at nonweight-bearing depths and limit activity to intensity levels below the onset of pain.[1] He or she would then progress to increased percentages of weight bearing and intensity levels as symptoms allowed. Specific

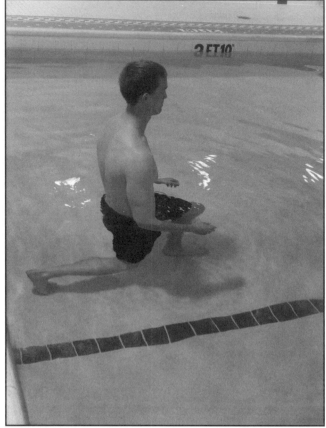

Figure 2-4. Lunge.

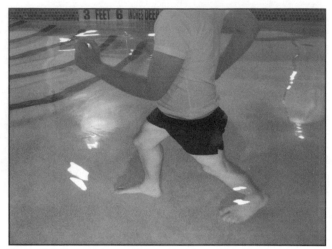

Figure 2-5. Deep water running.

exercises that can be used during aquatic therapy will be discussed in depth in subsequent chapters.

In addition to providing a variety of benefits for individuals rehabilitating from injuries to their upper and lower extremities, aquatic therapy is often indicated for the treatment of acute low back injuries or chronic low back pain. Therapy for low back pain focuses on whole-body exercises, core stabilization exercises, as well as exercises that target the spinal stabilizers (primarily the lumbar multifidi and transverse abdominus).[11] Ideal exercises are ones that maximize the activation of these muscles while minimizing the loads placed on the spine. The decreased loading on the vertebrae and traction forces that can be applied to the spine when performing exercises in the water can be of great value to these individuals. Additionally, floating supine in the water allows the lumbar spine to be placed in varying degrees of extension and hyperextension, which can provide symptomatic relief to individuals with herniated discs or with nerve root compression symptoms.[4] The spine is well protected during aquatic exercise,[1] and buoyancy can reduce spinal loads, as hydrostatic pressure and warm water assist in pain control and increased mobility.[11] Similar exercises for the treatment of low back pain that are performed on land can be performed in the water with equal benefit to the patient. Studies show that abdominal hallowing, pelvic tilts, and alternating arm and leg lift exercises are best when trying to achieve maximum activation

of the spinal stabilizers (lumbar multifidus and transverse abdominus) without activation of more superficial abdominal muscles (rectus abdominus and the obliques). However, if the goal of the exercise is to globally maximize activation of all trunk muscles, then abdominal bracing combined with exercises such as squats or lunges (Figure 2-4) and exercises involving the use of a physioball should be used.[11] Individuals with low back pain should participate in aquatic therapy that involves spinal stabilization techniques (Figure 2-5) along with an aerobic component.[1] Bressel et al found that aquatic therapy at the xyphoid process level depth in a temperature of 30°C, including exercises such as abdominal hollowing, abdominal bracing, pelvic tilts, physioball pushdowns, lateral pushdowns and rotations, hip abduction, stationary marching, and alternating arm raises in the transverse and sagittal planes, has been shown to improve symptoms in individuals with low back pain.[11]

AQUATIC THERAPY IN THE REHABILITATION OF ATHLETES

Aquatic therapy provides athletes with an excellent way to maintain their current fitness levels during the off-season or while rehabilitating from an injury. Hydrotherapy can be used to assist in off-loading a joint, allowing an injured athlete to keep up his or her fitness level and return to exercise without risk of further injury to or breakdown of the involved structures.[1,3] Studies that compared aquatic training to traditional land-based training found that injured athletes participating in aquatic therapy were able to regain function more rapidly than those participating in land-based therapy, especially during the early phases of rehabilitation.[5]

Aquatic therapy can be used for upper extremity, lower extremity, and core strengthening exercises as well as for neuromuscular reeducation via balance and proprioceptive activities.[3] Further, aquatic therapy is a useful cross-training technique that has been shown to be as effective at maintaining fitness levels as land-based training without adding additional joint forces.[1,8] In addition to standard strengthening exercises, injured athletes can practice sport-specific exercises by using buoyancy and resistance to their advantage. Therefore, athletes can restore functional capabilities and cardiovascular endurance sooner than they would if they participated solely in land-based therapy. Several cardiovascular benefits have been found in athletes training in water, such as improved athletic performance from inspiratory muscle training including improved ability to breathe during peak exercise levels when returning to land after aquatic exercise.[1]

Injured athletes can also partake in deep water running as a way of maintaining fitness levels or returning to running after an injury. Running movements of varying stride lengths and frequencies can be used to simulate running mechanics as well as to help strengthen hip and lower lumbar regions.[4] Additionally, evidence shows that deep water running can maintain the fitness level of an elite athlete for up to 6 weeks provided that he or she uses the same duration, frequency, and intensity at which he or she is accustomed to training.[4,8] Cross-country skiing performed in the water has also been shown to maintain fitness levels in athletes and is a nice alternative to deep water running for maintaining or increasing cardiovascular levels. Deep water running requires minimal ROM at the shoulder and a large ROM at the hips and knees and is an ideal cardiovascular training method for athletes with shoulder pathology or who participate in sports requiring larger ROMs of the lower extremity. Cross-country skiing, however, requires large ROM of the shoulders and hips but not of the knees and may be a preferred method of training for those with knee pathology.[3]

Athletes often need to recover and return to their sports as quickly as possible, and water provides an excellent environment in which to begin aggressive early functional rehabilitation with the lowest possibility of subsequent reinjury or aggravation of symptoms.[5] Athletes can use aquatic exercise during their off-season or when needing active rest because it allows them to maintain their high level of fitness while resting an injury.

AQUATIC THERAPY FOR INDIVIDUALS WITH OSTEOARTHRITIS

Aquatic therapy has been shown to improve quality of life, physical activity levels, pain, and muscle strength in individuals with osteoarthritis (OA).[6] Traditional land-based weight-bearing exercises often place too much stress on osteoarthritic joints, preventing individuals with OA from participating in exercise regimens. However, several of these exercises can be performed in the water, allowing these individuals to strengthen necessary muscles without increasing joint loading. Individuals with OA who participate in aquatic therapy are 12 times more likely to report global pain improvement compared to controls,[6] and improvements in impairments have been shown to last up to 6 weeks after resolution of a supervised aquatic therapy program.[6]

The buoyancy of water allows for decreased joint stresses and weight bearing through the lower extremities, which promotes a more pain-free way of exercising the necessary muscles than is available via traditional land-based therapy.[6] Additionally, warm water can help to reduce joint stiffness and muscle guarding, further reducing the stresses placed on joints.[6] Movement in water is often easier than on land, and individuals with OA can exercise with less effort and through a greater ROM than they otherwise would be able to.

In addition to the benefits already discussed, aquatic therapy has been shown to improve strength and flexibility in individuals with OA.[6,9] Decreased quadriceps strength is highly associated with increased levels of pain in individuals with knee OA,[6] and therefore quadriceps strengthening should be a main focus of any rehabilitation program either on land or in the water. The decreased joint forces and weight bearing that the properties of water provide allow for individuals with hip and knee OA to successfully complete more aggressive weight-bearing exercises for quadriceps strengthening than they would be able to on land. Additionally, increased knee and hip flexion strength and flexibility, which can be achieved from aquatic therapy, assist in increasing walking efficiency and decreasing disability associated with ADL in individuals with hip and knee OA.[9] The ability to participate in a wide variety of exercises also helps the self-efficacy and psychological well-being of these individuals and helps improve their adherence to the exercise program.[9]

An aquatic rehabilitation program for individuals with knee or hip OA should include exercises that focus on hip muscle and quad strengthening, as well as core stabilization, balance, and proprioception, because these exercises have been shown to be effective in decreasing the symptoms of OA.[12] Exercises should be performed in functional positions, and the resistance should be increased as tolerated by the patient's symptoms.[6] Exercises should also incorporate walking components to emphasize proper gait mechanics, which can often be lost as the disease progresses. One study found that exercising 3 times a week for 12 weeks with exercise sessions that lasted 50 to 60 min and focused on all major joints of the extremities as well as the trunk improved pain symptoms, strength, and flexibility in individuals with OA.[9] Aquatic therapy programs of moderate intensity can therefore be used to improve flexibility, upper and lower extremity strength, and aerobic fitness without further injury or deterioration of joint condition in individuals with OA.[9]

DESIGN OF EXERCISE PROGRAM

Several factors should be taken into consideration when designing an aquatic therapy program, including impairments, age of the patient, ultimate goals of the individual, and comfort level. No matter what the goal of the therapy session or which exercises are going to be focused on, all sessions should begin with a proper warm-up, such as walking, biking, or calisthenics, and end with a cool-down that includes stretching techniques.[3,5] Aquatic therapy aimed at maintaining or improving cardiovascular endurance can include deep water or hydrotrack running, cross-country skiing, waist-deep aqua running, or water cycling. General recommendations suggest exercising for 25 to 30 min a day 5 times a week to maintain cardiovascular fitness levels; however, elite athletes may require increased amounts of exercise.[3] Individuals can train at levels 17 to 20 bpm lower than their typical heart rate during exercise while still maintaining fitness levels because the maximum heart rate levels off during exercise in aquatic therapy.[3] Typical water temperatures of therapeutic pools are between 34°C and 35°C[5] but can be increased or decreased depending on the goal of the therapy session and the individual.

For athletes using aquatic therapy for rehabilitation or off-season training, exercises should be as sport specific as possible and can include aerobic conditioning, strength training, and plyometric drills to achieve the maximum level of carryover when returning to land-based exercise. For example, flutter kick exercises can be performed by those involved in sports requiring short forceful movements of the lower extremities or those requiring trunk stabilization.[3] As long as the aquatic therapy prescription is in line with the goals of the patient and keeps the restrictions of the underlying pathology in mind, aquatic therapy can be an ideal adjunct to land-based therapy.

AQUATIC THERAPY IN SPECIAL POPULATIONS

In addition to individuals with orthopedic injuries, aquatic therapy can provide numerous benefits to individuals suffering from cardiovascular disease as well as those with neurological impairments, rheumatic diseases, or chronic pain problems.

Cardiovascular Impairments

Individuals with cardiovascular impairments often benefit from an exercise program; however, many times they cannot participate in land-based therapy for a long enough duration or high enough intensity to improve upon their impairments. Aquatic therapy and water immersion cause several changes to the cardiovascular system that can be helpful for this population.[1,3] For individuals with poor cardiac output or ejection fractions, immersion in warm water can help improve both of these impairments. Warm water immersion can increase heart rate and thus cardiac output, with cardiac output increasing 1500 mL/min of clavicle depth immersion.[1,3] Fifty percent of this increase in cardiac output is increased blood muscle flow,[1,3] meaning that increased oxygen is being circulated to the muscles, allowing for longer exercise durations before becoming fatigued. Additionally, ejection fraction can increase as much as 30% with exercise in warm water environments, with a concomitant decrease in left ventricular end-diastolic volume.[1] Therefore, patients with very low ejection fractions who may not be able to participate in most traditional land-based therapies might experience greater success with aquatic therapy.

Patients with high blood pressure need to be closely monitored when exercising because systolic blood pressure increases with increasing workloads.[1] Though systolic blood pressure still increases with aquatic therapy, it is typically 20% less in water than on land,[1] providing a safer environment for these individuals to exercise in. For patients with cardiac disease resulting in higher-than-normal heart rates and cardiac output, aquatic therapy in colder water may be more beneficial. Immersion in colder water can decrease the heart rate by 12% to 15%, which decreases cardiac output.[1,3] If patients with higher-than-normal heart rates are going to participate in an exercise program at typical therapeutic pool temperatures, extra care should be taken to monitor their vital signs to ensure that they do not overexert themselves. Aquatic therapy with pool temperatures ranging from 31°C to 38°C has proved to be a safe and effective rehabilitation alternative for hypo-, hyper-, and normotensive individuals with cardiac impairments.[1]

Individuals with pulmonary impairments can use aquatic therapy as a type of pulmonary rehabilitation as well. Immersion in water affects the pulmonary system because immersion to the level of the thorax causes a shift in blood volume toward the chest cavity, resulting in greater compression on the chest wall due to the pressure of the water.[1] This increased pressure on the chest cavity results in increased work during normal respiration, with the majority of the increased work occurring during inspiration.[1] Patients with pulmonary dysfunction such as those with chronic obstructive pulmonary disease (COPD) or congestive heart failure can therefore use aquatic therapy as a form of inspiratory muscle training in addition to the regular aquatic strength training that has been discussed previously.[1] It is recommended that patients with COPD begin aquatic therapy at waist-deep levels to decrease the amount of pressure placed on the thorax and progress to deeper levels as their strength, respiratory capacity, and tolerance improve.[1]

Neurological Population

Individuals suffering from a variety of neurological diseases, such as those who have experienced a stroke or who have multiple sclerosis, amyotrophic lateral sclerosis, or spinal cord injuries, often have impairments such as hemiparesis, decreased balance, decreased proprioception, decreased ROM, and difficulty with ambulation. The physical properties of water, especially buoyancy, can allow individuals with these impairments to participate in a greater number of exercises without assistance and without the risk of falling or further injury.[10] Buoyancy allows for decreased weight bearing and reduces the effort needed to support the body.[10] A study by Noh et al in 2008 found that an 8-week-long aquatic therapy program for individuals who had experienced a stroke resulted in increased strength of the paretic leg in addition to improvements in balance, ability to rise from a chair, ability to transfer weight onto the affected side, and gait mechanics.[10] All of these improvements were despite the chronic nature of the disease. The aquatic therapy performed in the study consisted of an hour-long session in 34°C water including 10 min of light warm-up and 20 min of balance exercises in the transverse and sagittal planes as well as combined motions. This was followed by 20 min of balance training that focused mostly on the involved side and then ended with a 10-min cool-down.[10] Because individuals with neurological pathologies often have decreased cognitive function, extra care and attention needs to be used with this population, and one-on-one therapy sessions are often recommended.

Rheumatoid Arthritis

Rheumatoid arthritis (RA) is an autoimmune disorder that results in chronic inflammation of several joints of the body resulting in joint stiffness and decreased ROM. Despite the common feelings of warm, swollen joints, warm water aquatic therapy can be beneficial for individuals with RA.[7] Aquatic therapy can be used to increase overall joint flexibility and ROM using the techniques and properties of water previously discussed in this chapter. Increased ROM and flexibility are correlated with an improved functional status in this population.[7] Significant increases in active ROM into dorsiflexion, hip abduction, shoulder flexion, and elbow extension have been seen in individuals with RA who participate in aquatic therapy.[7] These improvements, along with decreased pain and difficulty completing ADL, lead to an increase in functional ability for this patient population.[7] When patients are experiencing acute joint symptoms, gentle active or active-assisted ROM activities in warm water are indicated; however, when the symptoms are more subacute or chronic, a more active exercise regimen is of greater benefit.[1,7] Aquatic therapy for these individuals should focus on motion of all of the major joints of the extremities and trunk, as well as isometric and isotonic exercises against the resistance of the water.[7] Aquatic therapy should be used in conjunction with typical treatments for this disease, such as controlled medication intake, monitoring of disease exacerbations and remissions, and improvement in work efficiency in order to optimally enhance the daily lives of individuals with RA.[7]

Fibromyalgia

Fibromyalgia is a chronic musculoskeletal pain disorder characterized by a variety of symptoms, such as fatigue, low muscle performance, sleep disturbance, anxiety, and cognitive dysfunction.[13] The increase in ROM and strength and decrease in pain that aquatic therapy can provide makes it an ideal rehabilitation choice for these individuals. Patients with fibromyalgia who participate in aquatic therapy have demonstrated improvements in pain, sleep quality, cognitive function, and physical fitness and have shown greater improvements that took place at a faster rate than would have occurred with land-based therapy.[13] Aquatic therapy can also improve endurance in these individuals as well as decrease their scores on the Fibromyalgia Impact Questionnaire, an outcome assessment that measures how much the disease impacts their daily life.[13] This population demonstrates good adherence to aquatic therapy, which is an essential component of any rehabilitation or exercise program.[13] Aquatic therapy sessions should take place in warmer water temperatures at chest height depth. Sessions should include a warm-up and cool-down and focus on strengthening and aerobic exercises performed at 50% to 80% of age-adjusted predicted maximum heart rate.[13] As with an aquatic therapy program for individuals with RA, if the symptoms are more acute, gentler active or active-assisted exercises are recommended, whereas if the symptoms are more subacute or chronic, more aggressive exercises are safe and of more benefit to improve symptoms.[1]

Geriatric Population

Several impairments arise as a result of the general aging process, such as decreased strength, endurance, ROM, flexibility, and gait mechanics. Aquatic therapy can offer a safe environment for the geriatric population to improve upon these without the fear of falling or experiencing a debilitating injury.[1] Aquatic therapy has also been shown to improve the reaction time, movement speed, functional fitness, strength, endurance, and flexibility of geriatric patients, which can all lead to an overall improvement in psychological well-being.[1] Despite the decreased weight bearing experienced by individuals when performing exercises in the water, general musculoskeletal impairments can improve in individuals with osteoporosis and some studies demonstrate that aquatic therapy can even result in a decrease in incidence of falls; however, there is still equivocal evidence to support this claim.[1]

Bariatric Population

Traditional land-based therapy is often difficult for the bariatric population not only because of safety considerations associated with guarding this population but also because of the increased effort and stress to the joints that are involved in active ROM and resistance exercises. With aquatic therapy, body weight can be reduced to almost nothing, allowing this population to work on restoring fitness levels, since they are able to exercise for long enough periods of time to experience a training effect.[1] The buoyancy of water minimizes joint stresses and therefore decreases potential injuries to joints that can occur with land-based exercise.[1] Additionally, the thermal conductive properties of water allow bariatric patients to exercise for longer durations without risk of overheating, especially when exercising in water temperatures slightly cooler than typical therapeutic pools (below 34°C).[1] Aquatic therapy for this population should take place in slightly cooler water temperatures at a depth of about chest level and should consist of general ROM and strengthening exercises as well as sustained aerobic conditioning, balance, and coordination drills.[1]

Prenatal

Exercise is encouraged for pregnant women, and aquatic therapy offers a safe and effective alternative form of exercise for this population. Conventional pool temperatures have been shown to be safe during all trimesters of pregnancy, and aquatic therapy can assist with aerobic conditioning while decreasing joint loading.[1] Prenatal women are very sensitive to any increase in core body temperature, thus reducing the potential for overheating. With this in mind, however, it is still recommended that prenatal women limit their time of immersion in water temperatures of greater than or equal to 40°C to 15 min or less.[1] Neutral or cooler temperature pools are preferred with this population, and aquatic therapy should focus on general aerobic conditioning and strengthening with particular focus on spinal stabilizers, as low back pain is a common impairment in this population.[1]

SAFETY CONSIDERATIONS

Basic safety is important in all aspects of rehabilitation. The next chapter will discuss environmental considerations and how to choose the appropriate team to participate in the development of an aquatic therapy rehabilitation program; however, proper safety, precautions, and absolute contraindications for participation in an aquatic rehabilitation program will briefly be laid out here.

Entering and Exiting the Pool

The patient must have the ability to enter and exit the pool safely, either independently or with assistance, in order for aquatic therapy to be a viable option. In many cases, this lack of access may limit the initiation of therapy. If a lift is not available or the patient exceeds the weight limits of the lift, the patient will have to enter and exit via stairs. This may not be possible for patients with extreme muscle weakness, weight-bearing restrictions, or limitations. In

this case, if ramp access is available, the patient may enter using a wheelchair.

Comfort in Water

Fear of water may be a concern for a number of appropriate candidates. The patient should have a moderate level of comfort in the pool to participate or an unsafe environment could be created for both the patient and therapist. Patients should tolerate having their face in the water and be able to participate in rhythmic breathing or bobbing. In addition, it is helpful if the patient is able to float supine and prone with the ability to recover to a vertical position. Patients with a relative discomfort may benefit from a pool with handrails, additional supports, minimal to no turbulence, and low staff-to-client ratio. If aerobic conditioning is the main focus of the aquatic therapy program, a hydrotrack can be a good alternative to a therapy pool. If initiating an aquatic therapy program with an individual who has a fear of water, begin at a lower depth of water as long as he or she can tolerate the commensurate amount of weight bearing.

Postoperative Considerations

Immediate postoperative care usually focuses on prevention of deep vein thrombosis, wound healing, and protected ROM and weight bearing. As discussed previously, many of the properties of aquatic therapy make it an ideal environment for early postoperative care for both lower and upper extremity injuries. Despite the many benefits, aquatic therapy is often not introduced postoperatively, with access often being the primary reason. Postoperative patients with weight-bearing limitations must have access to a pool with a ramp or lift in order to participate. In addition, consideration should be taken to protect the surgical site and avoid any complications. In order for the postoperative patient to be a candidate, there should not be any doubt regarding postoperative complications, including the presence or risk of deep vein thrombosis, difficulty breathing, or uncontrolled blood pressure. The surgical site must also be clear of infection and bleeding and any wounds or incisions covered with a 100% occlusive, waterproof dressing.[14]

Wounds

Surgical wounds need to be covered with an occlusive, waterproof dressing.[14] These dressings are usually made of fine, transparent, elastic, self-adhering polyurethane film. The materials are nonporous, making them water- and bacteria-proof. In addition, these materials are flexible, allowing them to be applied directly over the joint (ie, post–total knee replacement) allowing free movement so as not to hinder the exercises being initiated. Pre-immersion, the surrounding area must be dry for the dressing to adhere and for the wound to remain moist. This prevents the dressing from adhering directly to the wound and prevents the new cells from being destroyed upon removal of the dressing. Postimmersion, the dressing should be removed immediately, the surrounding tissue dried, and an appropriate dressing reapplied if necessary.

Precautions and Absolute Contraindications

A number of relative precautions must be considered when initiating an aquatic program with a patient. The majority of absolute contraindications for an aquatic-based program are similar to those for land-based programs and consist of issues that would put the patient or therapist at risk. If the patient is medically unstable, exercise both on land and in water are contraindicated. Table 2-1 lays out which conditions require precaution and screening prior to initiation of an aquatic therapy program and which are contraindications to aquatic therapy.

CONCLUSION

The ultimate goal of any rehabilitation is a return to the patient's desired level of functional activity, return to recreational or sports activities, or merely a return to independent completion of activities of daily living. Ideally, a rehabilitation program should attempt to accomplish this while preventing reinjury and assuring proper healing of involved structures. Aquatic therapy provides a unique environment in which this can be achieved, because it promotes normal movement patterns and often increases strength and ROM earlier in a course of treatment than land-based exercise can.[4] These improvements are achieved in a setting that is safe in terms of its ability to protect the injured structure as well as reduce the risk of loss of balance or falls. Aquatic therapy is also frequently associated with reduced feelings of pain and perceived discomfort[4] and is helpful as an adjunct or precursor to land-based therapy. In certain situations, however, aquatic therapy may be the only solution for individuals for which traditional land-based rehabilitation is not an option or has not worked.

REFERENCES

1. Becker BE. Aquatic therapy: scientific foundations and clinical rehabilitation applications. *PM R.* 2009;1:859–872.
2. Prentice WE. *Athletic Training.* 11th ed. New York: McGraw-Hill; 2003.
3. Thein JM, Brody LT. Aquatic-based rehabilitation and training for the elite athlete. *J Orthop Sports Phys Ther.* 1998;27:32–41.
4. Prins J, Cutner D. Aquatic therapy in the rehabilitation of athletic injuries. *Clin Sports Med.* 1999;18:447–461.
5. Kim E, Kim T, Kang H, Lee J, Childers MK. Aquatic versus land-based exercises as early functional rehabilitation for elite athletes with acute lower extremity ligament injury: a pilot study. *PM R.* 2010;2:703–712.
6. Hinman RS, Heywood SE, Day AR. Aquatic physical therapy for hip and knee osteoarthritis: results of a single-blind randomized controlled trial. *Phys Ther.* 2007;87:32–43.
7. Templeton MS, Booth DL, O'Kelly WD. Effects of aquatic therapy on joint flexibility and functional ability in subjects with rheumatic disease. *J Orthop Sports Phys Ther.* 1996;23:376–381.
8. Kilgore GL. Deep-water running: a practical review of the literature with an emphasis on biomechanics. *Phys Sportsmed.* 2012;40:116–126.
9. Wang TJ, Belz B, Elaine Thompson F, Whitney JD, Bennett K. Effects of aquatic exercise on flexibility, strength, and aerobic fitness in adults with osteoarthritis of the hip or knee. *J Adv Nurs.* 2007;57:141–152.
10. Noh DK, Lim JY, Shin HI, Paik NJ. The effect of aquatic therapy on postural balance and muscle strength in stroke survivors—a randomized controlled pilot trial. Clin Rehabil. 2008;22:966–976.
11. Bressel E, Doiny DG, Vandenberg C, Cronin JB. Trunk muscle activity during spine stabilization exercises performed in a pool. *Phys Ther Sport.* 2012;13(2):67–72.
12. Bartels EM, Lund H, Hagen KB, Dagfinrund H, Christensen R, Danneskiold-Samsøe B. Aquatic exercise for the treatment of knee and hip osteoarthritis. *Cochrane Database Syst Rev.* 2007;17(4):CD005523.
13. Munguía-Izquierda D, Legaz-Arrese A. Assessment of the effects of aquatic therapy on global symptomology in patients with fibromyalgia syndrome: a randomized controlled trial. *Arch Phys Med Rehabil.* 2008;89:2250–2257.
14. Larsen J, Pryce M, Harrison J, et al. *Guidelines for Physiotherapists Working in and/or Managing Hydrotherapy Pools.* Victoria, Australia: Australian Physiotherapy Association; 2002.

Table 2-1.

Indications and Contraindications for Aquatic Therapy

System/Condition	Precautions/Screening	Contraindication
Cardiovascular	Unstable cardiac conditions High/low blood pressure Peripheral vascular disease	
Respiratory	Chronic and acute disease Shortness of breath at rest or on exertion Decreased vital capacity Tracheostomy	
Central nervous system	Epilepsy (treat one on one) Swallowing difficulties High dependency individuals	
Gastrointestinal	Colostomies	Fecal incontinence Uncontrolled diarrhea or gastroenteritis (no entering of pool for 7 to 10 days after resolution of symptoms)
Genitourinary	Menstruation Pregnancy	Urinary incontinence Bladder infections Pregnancy with bleeding
Integumentary	Surgical wounds External fixators Altered sensation Chlorine/bromine allergy (check which type of pool) Plantar warts	Skin grafts that have not completely healed Open wounds Active infection Tinea (ringworm) Infected skin rashes Wounds not covered with 100% occlusive dressing
Auditory/visual	Visual impairment Hearing impairment Contact lenses Tubal implants	
Infections		Diseases with airborne particles such as active tuberculosis, flu, or viral infections Herpes simplex with sores present
Other	Acute inflammatory conditions Heat-sensitive conditions limit time in warmer water temperatures ($< 34°C$) Radiotherapy (careful monitoring of patient's skin) Fear of water Cognitive impairments Behavioral disorders	

Adapted from Larsen J, Pryce M, Harrison J, et al. *Guidelines for Physiotherapists Working in and/or Managing Hydrotherapy Pools.* Victoria, Australia: Australian Physiotherapy Association; 2002.

3

Pool Selection, Facility Design, and Engineering Considerations

David M. Joyner, MD, FACS and Anson J. Flake, Esq

In the United States alone, there are approximately 270,000 commercial pools that are used for recreation, swimming, rehabilitation, and sports activities daily.[1] These commercial pools vary considerably in their specific design, and the aquatic facilities they are located within are vastly different from one another. In this book, we are primarily focused on the utilization of aquatics for orthopedic rehabilitation and conditioning, so we will keep our discussion to pools and facility design issues that we see in those orthopedic rehabilitation and conditioning environments.

CHOOSING YOUR FACILITY'S AQUATIC DESIGN

The design and configuration of any aquatic-based orthopedic, hospital, sports medicine, or physical therapy facility should endeavor to include the collaborative efforts of the administration or owners of the facility; the doctors, physical therapists, and athletic trainers prescribing and providing the aquatic therapy services to patients or athletes; and, in most cases, an experienced aquatic design consultant or architect. This integrated design approach assures that the space is functional, safe, and aesthetically pleasing to all of the stakeholders involved in the project. In this section, we will explore best practices to achieve these goals.

Integrating Your Aquatic Mission Within the Design of the Facility

The first step is to assess your available physical space, budget, and primarily your mission and goals for your aquatic orthopedic facility. Are your goals to have your patient or athlete population treated as a large group in the pool? Or is the goal to have a more intimate, "1-to-1" or "1-to-4" therapist to patient(s) type of pool setting? Is this a stand-alone pool facility or is the aquatic facility physically attached to an orthopedic practice, sports stadium, training center, or physical therapy clinic and needs to offer a connected and seamless traffic pattern for the aquatic users? Do you plan to offer both aquatic therapy and sports performance training in your aquatic facility? These types of questions are critical to ask well before you begin choosing the functional design elements of the facility or selecting the aquatic therapy pool or you might find yourself pursuing a design that is counterproductive to your desired objectives. No one wins in that scenario.

Once you have answered your overall mission questions and the goals are established and on paper, you are ready to consider your pool design and functionality. As mentioned in the opening remarks of this section, it is highly recommended that you foster a collaborative design approach to your aquatic space layout as well as the choice of your pool. By this, we mean to say that you should bring together

Wilk KE, Joyner DM. *The Use of Aquatics in Orthopedic and Sports Medicine Rehabilitation and Physical Conditioning (pp 27-33).*

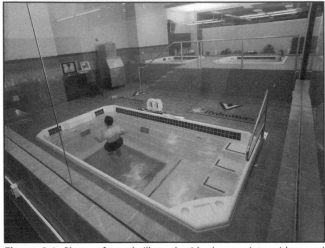

Figure 3-1. Photo of treadmill pool with therapy jets, video, and elevated hot and cold plunges at athletic medicine center. (Reprinted with permission from HydroWorx).

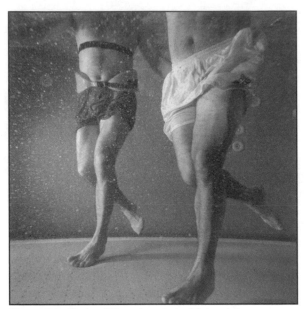

Figure 3-2. Photo of 2 postsurgical athletes doing crossover steps on a large underwater treadmill system.

the owners, administration, athletic trainers, or clinicians using the pool facility day to day and a reputable aquatic consultant or architect with experience in aquatic design. This type of collaboration gives the aquatic stakeholders an opportunity to express design and pool functionality concerns within the feedback loop of the aquatic design consultant or architect. When these stakeholders have tied down the wants and desires in terms of budget, function, space, and time frames for construction and tied those objectives fluently to the overall aquatic mission of the organization, you are now properly poised to achieve an exceptional design and pool selection process.

Selecting the Right Therapy and Conditioning Pool for You

There are a handful of key questions that you may want to ask yourself in preparing to go through the process of selecting the aquatic therapy pool to put in your facility: First, per our established mission and goals for the overall facility, what types of conditions or activities do we wish to treat in our pool? Second, how many athletes or patients do we plan to treat throughout the typical workday? Third, how many patients or athletes do we wish to treat at any one time so that the quality of care is consistent with our mission and goals? These questions, and more, when answered after careful analysis, will help cultivate a thoughtful selection process of the appropriate therapy and conditioning pool for your application.

Two Primary Types of Pools to Consider

There are 2 primary types of pools used for aquatic rehabilitation and conditioning in the orthopedic field today and they are significantly different in their function, design, size, and even the outcomes that can be achieved from their use. In the first instance, we have the smaller, highly functional and technologically advanced therapy and conditioning pool or machine (Figure 3-1). This type of pool is often referred to as a water therapy or aquatic therapy machine due to its advanced technological design. The top manufacturers of these pools offer underwater treadmill systems (Figure 3-2) and moveable floors that act like water-based elevators, transporting patients and athletes safely to any desired depth for rehab or conditioning. Additionally, they may include underwater video monitoring systems and powerful jet systems for deep tissue massage and resistance exercises. All of these advanced features are conveniently linked to a sophisticated software and computer system to track progress and provide visual underwater video feedback for the user and the clinician.

These therapeutic water machines are typically in an 8-ft × 12-ft format but some have been built as large as 12 ft × 16 ft. They are designed to treat from 4 to 8 patients or athletes at any given time and can provide a host of billable aquatic therapy modalities.

The highly functional aquatic therapy pools offer the clinician and his or her user population specific rehabilitation and conditioning activities that translate directly to land-based activities. As an example, a patient may use an underwater treadmill system for gait training, therapeutic exercise, plyometrics, and sports performance activities in the water. These upright water exercises reflect what patients and athletes typically do on land and that is an important feature of these types of pools. In America, fewer than 5% of the population can swim 400 yards without stopping, but 98% can walk vertically in the water, and this fact reinforces the impact of these smaller, functional pools for the majority of the population who run or sprint upright on land.[2]

Moreover, when land-specific upright water rehabilitation is combined with diagnostic visual feedback from the underwater video camera system and at a user body weight of only 10% of their land body weight, one has the opportunity to achieve aggressive rehab or training outcomes.[3]

Eventually, this patient or athlete progresses to land-based activities where he or she engages in nearly the same activities he or she was doing in the water but now with his or her full body weight in play.

The second choice for an aquatic therapy pool is to consider a larger, more traditional community or lap pool design (Figure 3-3). This type of pool is generally colder than the smaller therapy pool and is not as technologically advanced. However, it offers the advantage of treating more patients or athletes at any given time. Aerobic classes and group treatment sessions can be conducted in this type of pool easily.

Additionally, when not being used for therapy purposes, the community type of pool is often converted into a swimming pool and swim classes and training are offered. These broad uses give this type of pool additional diversity that can be effective to meet an aquatic mission that asks for a large patient or athlete population.

It is apparent that each type of pool design offers unique characteristics for therapy and conditioning clinicians to choose between. To aid that selection process, Table 3-1 presents the most frequently used options, designs, and advantages and limitations of each type of pool.

Architectural, Engineering, and Construction Considerations

Once you have selected the pool system that fits your aquatic mission, the next step is to engage your architect, athletic trainers, clinicians, and administrators and integrate the chosen therapy pool into your specific aquatic facility design. There are many steps in this stage of planning and design, and the sections that follow are highlighted to make you aware of many of the key areas to consider.

Federal, State, and Local Codes

Because regulatory and code requirements vary significantly from state to state, and even between local jurisdictional agencies, permitting and compliance with state and local provisions relative to health, pool and spa, building, electrical, plumbing, mechanical, and safety is a key responsibility of the owner. Therefore, it is critical that the owner and/or his authorized architect or aquatic design consultant engage the appropriate pool and spa agencies

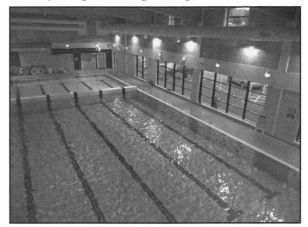

Figure 3-3. Photo of large lap pool or community-style pool.

at the local and state level to ensure compliance with the applicable regulatory requirements.

The Occupational Safety and Health Administration (OSHA) is also tasked with regulating pools. Three OSHA regulations should be considered when planning your aquatic facility: OSHA 29 CFR 1910.1200: Hazard Communications Standard[4]; OSHA 29 CFR 1910.146: Confined Spaces Regulation[5]; and OSHA 29 CFR 1910.1030: Occupational Exposure to Blood Borne Pathogens.[6] Additionally, as of December 1, 2008, a new federal law was enacted: the Virginia Graeme Baker Pool and Spa Safety Act,[7] whose overall mission is to reduce the child drowning and suction entrapment incidents, injuries, and deaths in both residential and public pools. It requires that all pool or spa drain covers sold after December 19, 2008, must meet ASME/ANSI A112.19.8–2007. If your therapy or conditioning pool is regulated and is defined by your state as a public pool, this standard applies to you and you must comply.[8]

It is imperative to contact the pool supplier you have selected immediately should regulatory or code circumstance arise requiring variation in the therapy pool design.

A copy of your state's codes can be downloaded from the National Swimming Pool Foundation Web site at www.nspf.org.

Access and Service of the Pool and Equipment

Architectural, structural, mechanical, electrical, and plumbing design criteria identified by the pool designer or the pool manufacturer must be maintained for future serviceability of the pool and its pumps, filters, drains, and all equipment. Not adhering to these pool design requirements may result in poor routine service and, in the worst cases, the manufacturer voiding the product's warranty.

Site Preparation

In most cases, the pool owner is responsible for the cost and preparation of the site prior to the pool installation.

Table 3-1.

Advantages and Limitations of Pool Types Used in Orthopedic Rehabilitation and Conditioning Settings

	Smaller, Technologically Advanced Style Pools	**Larger Lap or Community-Style Pools**
Design	• Typically warm water, 88°F to 94°F • Typically 2.5 to 6.0 ft deep, even bottom or gradual slope or moveable floor • Often ground-level design • Usually small, designed away from large group treatment • Moveable floors, chair lifts, or ramp access most common • Smaller facility allocation needed for smaller pool footprint • Integrated treadmills and lift systems may require mechanical pit space	• Ground level • Cooler water, 82°F to 86°F • Usually ladders, ramps, or stair access; chair lifts in some circumstances • Varying sloped floor depths, typically 3 to 9 ft • Heavy occupancy
Advantages	• Advanced integrated technology such as treadmills, video, jets, and massage • Biomechanically correct walking or running gait via underwater treadmill • Unlimited water depth with moveable floor/adjustable water depth systems • Access to the pool via the moveable floor makes patient treatment safer • Progressive loading capabilities via the moveable floor/water depth system • Warm water more comfortable for activities and prolonged immersion • Ease of access for even severely disabled or paralyzed patients • Biomechanical feedback with underwater video assists in diagnostic coaching • Vertical and horizontal exercise options both feasible options against jets • Intense, high-pressure massage via jets and massage hoses	• Sloping floor and depth make broad range of program options feasible • Ideal for swimming and general conditioning/rehab programs • Vertical and horizontal options feasible

(continued)

All utilities (power, water, sanitary, etc) that are required for safe and reliable pool operation should be provided and installed by the owner per the construction or remodeling schedule.

Pool Room Design

The water treatment area of the pool room itself should be designed to safely and effectively accommodate the number of patients or athletes outlined in your aquatic mission and goals. One should closely follow state codes regarding the recommended minimum dimensions for the pool room and allowing adequate installation and deck space around the pool. Additional space may be required for dehumidification systems, cabinetry, storage, showers, changing rooms, and the like. Floor or perimeter drains must be incorporated into the design of the pool area. If

Table 3-1. (continued)

Advantages and Limitations of Pool Types Used in Orthopedic Rehabilitation and Conditioning Settings

	Smaller, Technologically Advanced Style Pools	Larger Lap or Community-Style Pools
Limitations	• Limited public access is typical • High temperature, if in place, may restrict use for advanced conditioning	• Lack of advanced technology limits functional rehab/performance use • Gait patterns are biomechanically compromised due to static pool floor • Biofeedback limited for clinician/patient for lack of underwater monitoring • Ease of water depth adjustment is limited in many cases • Cool water makes it difficult to stay warm during low-level activities • Challenging rehab environment for the severely disabled or paralyzed
Suitable populations	• Hospital-based acute rehabilitation • Joint replacement, other orthopedic populations • Neurological rehabilitation and acute paralysis patients • Sports team and sports medicine clinic injury rehabilitation • Sports-specific performance training • Arthritis and arthoplasty rehabilitation • Rehabilitation programs for deconditioned people • Obesity and weight loss programs	• Joint replacement, other orthopedic populations • General injury rehabilitation • Generalized sports performance training • Arthritis and arthoplasty rehabilitation • Rehabilitation programs for deconditioned people • Obesity and weight loss programs • Preventative conditioning programs for the healthy

Reprinted with permission from *Comprehensive Aquatic Therapy*, 3rd ed, published by Washington State University Publishing, Bruce E. Becker, MD and Andrew J. Cole, MD, Eds. ©2010, ISBN 978-0-615-36567-1.

floor drains are chosen, several should be placed around the pool with special attention to the high-traffic areas.

Adequate airflow, temperature control, and dehumidification in the pool room are required to maintain a comfortable temperature for the occupants and to protect against adverse conditions inherent with a humid environment. Pool rooms are typically kept at 82°F to 85°F to keep the variance between the pool water and the ambient air temperature at a minimum. In smaller, highly functional therapy pools, the anticipated daily pool evaporation rate under these conditions is approximately 15 to 20 gallons per day.

If the pool includes a computer, a control pendant, or an underwater video system and flat screen monitors, then the pool room must include cabinetry located in front of the pool to accommodate these components and the distance from the water's edge to any electrical equipment needs to exceed 10 ft in most cases (check your local and state codes to verify their exact distance requirements).

Mechanical Pit Surrounding the Pool

If a functional, smaller therapy pool is chosen, the mechanical pit design around the pool structure must include adequate access to the pool tank, accessory equipment (filter, pumps, heater, etc), and the electrical control panel. Recommended minimum dimensions for the mechanical pit must also include HVAC controls appropriate for the area, lighting, and a sump pump or drains in case of a pool leak or plumbing failure.

A pool's structural weight can be significant, and when combined with the pool's water weight (based around the number of gallons in the pool), this weight will be bearing on the mechanical pit floor; therefore, a structural engineer should be consulted to determine structural requirements for the mechanical pit floor.

The mechanical pit should be designed to maintain an ambient temperature typical for mechanical room occupancy during maintenance of the pool equipment. Analysis of equipment specs may be utilized for determining heat discharge and finalizing the appropriate HVAC design for the mechanical pit. You will want to analyze the following:

- Electric heater (or natural gas or propane)
- Horsepower of the therapy jet pump (if selected for the pool model chosen)
- Horsepower of the treadmill motor (if selected for the pool model chosen)
- Horsepower of the floor lift motor (if selected for the pool model chosen)
- Horsepower of the maintenance pump

Utilities

The following points will help clarify 4 often overlooked areas in mechanical pit and mechanical design that relate to utilities and communication.

- Water supply: The owner should provide a water supply line with an anti-siphon device connected to the circulation system as shown in the aquatic design drawings.
- Electrical service: The owner should provide electrical service drops designed for the requirements of the therapy pool's electrical control cabinet and separately for the heater.
- Sanitary: The owner should provide a sump pit with pump or floor drains for connection to the pool's maintenance system and main drains. The sanitary system should be designed to accommodate the total gallons of the pool via gravity flow.
- Communications: A telephone line located in close proximity to the pool's equipment for communication during system maintenance is always a good idea.

DESIGN AND CONSTRUCTION CHECKLIST

This checklist is designed to stimulate proactive design and construction coordination between all of the stakeholders on your project. It will help to assure that the pool is properly incorporated into the design and construction phase of your aquatic facility project.

- **Planning Question 1:** Have you had a design and coordination meeting with all of the design and construction representatives to discuss the overall aquatic mission, space design goals, scope of work, lessons learned, pool selected, etc? *This is critical to have as early as possible in the project. It is useful in understanding the connection between architectural, structural, mechanical, electrical, plumbing, and the design and installation requirements of your selected pool.*

- **Planning Question 2:** Have you requested AutoCAD files for the specific pool model that was selected by the owner so it can be properly integrated into the facility design? *The structural stage is not too early because these units have design requirements that significantly impact that phase of design.*

- **Planning Question 3:** Have you requested and incorporated the Construction Specification Institute (CSI) specs into the construction bid documents before the document goes to bid? *It is important to include the CSI specs for your pool and project details into the bid document because once it is out to bid, it is often too late to make changes and your project may end up incomplete or inadequate.*

- **Planning Question 4:** Have you provided the pool manufacturer or provider with the overall pool facility design for review and comment? *This is important as you want to be able to let the manufacturer of the pool comment on its integration into the mechanical, plumbing, and electrical design and how the pool is integrated into the overall aquatic facility design. This is a key step that is often overlooked.*

- **Planning Question 5:** Have you provided the pool manufacturer or provider with the project's approved final drawings? *The final drawings for the facility and pool room design need to be sent to the pool manufacturer so a final review can take place before you begin construction. It is more costly and it may delay the project if you fail to catch design issues until after you have begun construction. A final design review by the manufacturer can help prevent problems.*

- **Planning Question 6:** Have you submitted your aquatic facility design and pool design to the local and/or state health department for approval? *This is a key responsibility of the owner's representatives and is often left to the very end of a project; in some cases, code* *issues surface during the final occupancy process, which creates last-minute change orders so that the pool or the aquatic facility may become compliant with local, state, or federal codes.*

- **Planning Question 7:** Have you clarified the scope of work for the plumbing, electrical, and mechanical trades in the bid documents or the construction contracts? *Sometimes this results in change orders that impact the owner's design and his or her financial budget.*

- **Planning Question 8:** Have you adhered to the setback requirements for the service of the pool's equipment in the mechanical pit or equipment room? *Missing these setback requirements often leads to component failures due to incorrect design and lack of ventilation. This is a major problem seen on many therapy pool projects.*

- **Planning Question 9:** Have you designed for adequate air circulation in the mechanical pit or equipment mechanical room to address heat loads of equipment? *The motors and electronics located in the pool's mechanical pit needs to have adequate circulation and air flow to prevent overheating and costly service issues. It is important to have your architect design specifically for the heat load tolerances of all the equipment located in the pool's mechanical pit.*

- **Planning Question 10:** For prefabricated pools, have you confirmed the access route for the pool and all of its components so that the delivery sequencing at the job site flows seamlessly and without delay? *It is generally the architect and general contractor's responsibility to provide and maintain the required access route for the pool and its equipment from the point of delivery to the final installation location. This may require wall sections being left open, lintels or headers being used to maintain access, or possibly even roof sections being left open. The access plan for the pool and components must be reviewed with the pool manufacturer and the contractor throughout the project.*

- **Planning Question 11:** Have you seen the language, "Verify/coordinate with pool manufacturer"? It is a common note on architectural or engineering drawings that go to bid and its ambiguity leads to errors and omissions or change orders that can be avoided by verifying the design requirements precisely up front in the bid document. *The pool manufacturer should be involved early in the design and development phase of the aquatic facility project given the structural and foundation impacts of many therapy pools and the investment that the owner is making in the overall aquatic facility itself.*

- **Planning Question 12:** Have you sized the filtration, water chemistry, and circulation equipment to accommodate peak bather loads? *This is often miscalculated and results in cloudy or unsafe water conditions. This is critical and should be analyzed with the assistance of both the pool manufacturer and an aquatic consultant.*

CONCLUSION

Designing your aquatic facility for orthopedic rehabilitation and conditioning is best done when it is a collaborative approach between the facility owners, architects, aquatic consultant, and most importantly the physicians, athletic trainers, physical therapists, and strength and conditioning coaches. It is this team of professionals, working together, that will ensure selecting the right aquatic design and pool to satisfy the orthopedic rehabilitation mission.

A collaborative approach will ensure that all options have been considered and that the most appropriate pool has been seamlessly designed into the overall aquatic facility design. Endeavor to use experienced aquatic consultants and manufacturers to implement your design objectives in a proactive manner. Ask for and use "design and construction checklists" to ensure that all proactive design and architectural steps are being taken on the front end of the design process to create a successful and highly effective aquatic environment for your athletes, patients, and sports medicine team.

REFERENCES

1. Salzman A. Media statistics: how popular is aquatic therapy? Aquatic Resources Network site. http://www.aquaticnet.com/media-statistics.htm. Accessed August 2011.

2. Popke M. Aquatic exercise targets younger demographics. *Athletic Business.* May 2010. http://www.athleticbusiness.com/articles/article.aspx?articleid=3535&zoneid=6. Accessed August 2011

3. Salazar A, Dolny D. *Underwater Treadmill Running: The Low Impact, Pain Free, Calorie-Burning Fitness Advantage.* Middletown, PA: HydroWorx; 2012.

4. Occupational Safety & Health Administration, United States Department of Labor. Hazard Communications [Standard 1910.1200]. http://www.osha.gov/pls/oshaweb/owadisp.show_document?p_table=standards&p_id=10099. Accessed May 30, 2013.

5. Occupational Safety & Health Administration, United States Department of Labor. Permit-required confined spaces [Standard 1910.146]. http://www.osha.gov/pls/oshaweb/owadisp.show_document?p_table=standards&p_id=9797. Accessed May 30, 2013.

6. Occupational Safety & Health Administration, United States Department of Labor. Bloodborne pathogens [Standard 1910.1030]. http://www.osha.gov/pls/oshaweb/owadisp.show_document?p_table=standards&p_id=10051. Accessed May 30, 2013.

7. United States Consumer Product Safety Commission. Virginia Graeme Baker Pools and Spa Safety Act. http://www.poolsafely.gov/wp-content/uploads/pssa.pdf. Accessed May 30, 2013.

8. Osinski A. Facility design and water management. In: Becker BE, Cole AJ, eds. *Comprehensive Aquatic Therapy.* 3rd ed. Pullman: Washington State University Publishing; 2010:465–467.

Section II

Postinjury, Intervention, and Treatments

Aquatic Application for the Lower Extremity

Todd R. Hooks, PT, DMT, OCS, SCS, ATC, MOMT, MTC, CSCS, FAAOMPT;
Kevin E. Wilk, PT, DPT, FAPTA; and Jason Palmer, BHMS (Ed) Hons, BPhty, MCSP

Traditionally, the treatment and rehabilitation of lower limb injuries has been conducted in the hospital or clinic environment. Water, however, and the technological advances in therapy delivery, offers an alternative physical environment that can benefit the patient in many ways and can contribute significantly to the delivery of a comprehensive rehabilitation program.

When deciding whether a patient could benefit from an aquatic therapy program, consideration needs to be given to the patient's comfort with being partially submerged in water and the potential therapeutic benefits of the physical properties of water, which include the unloading of joints through buoyancy, hydrostatic pressure, water temperature, and viscosity. In addition to the physical properties of water, important technological advancements have been made in the past 2 decades, such as pools with integrated underwater treadmills, variable-speed resistance jets, hydro-massage hoses, support bars, adjustable floor depth, and underwater video systems that provide greater opportunities and advantages for the patient and therapist or athletic trainer. Therefore, most diagnoses could benefit from aquatic therapy when taking into consideration any possible contraindications.

Some common conditions at the ankle and foot that can benefit from therapy in the water include arthritis, fractures, inversion and eversion ankle sprains, syndesmotic ankle sprain, and tendinopathies (eg, Achilles tendonitis, plantar fasciitis, postsurgical tendon repairs, lateral ankle reconstructions).

Common conditions at the knee joint that can benefit from aquatic therapy include arthritis, fractures, meniscal injury, ligament sprain, chondral injuries, and muscle strains (eg, hamstring). In addition, postsurgical rehabilitation for conditions such as total knee replacement and anterior cruciate ligament (ACL) reconstruction also could significantly benefit from aquatic therapy.

Common conditions at the hip joint that can benefit from aquatic therapy include arthritis, bursitis, fractures, hip dislocations, hip flexor or adductor strains, as well as postoperative rehabilitation following total hip replacement or acetabular labral repair.

In this chapter we have included several treatment protocols in the appendices to help facilitate the utilization of aquatic therapy and more effectively treat the patient. These protocols include ACL rehab (Appendix A), rehabilitation following microfracture surgery (Appendix B), and rehabilitation following total hip and knee replacement (Appendices C, D, and E).

REHABILITATION GUIDELINES

Patients with various lower extremity pathologies constitute a large percentage of the population who are prescribed and benefit from aquatic therapy in traditional pool environments. On land, ground reaction forces and therefore joint and tissue loading vary depending upon the activity performed, ranging from 3.4 times body weight with level walking to 33 times body weight with running.[1-3] During weight-bearing activities, the lower extremity works as one functional unit and undergoes rhythmic loading; therefore, coordination of the lower limb joints is an essential part of lower limb rehabilitation. Water provides an excellent medium to nurture and regain these coordinated movements in a safe and supportive environment. For example,

Wilk KE, Joyner DM. *The Use of Aquatics in Orthopedic and Sports Medicine Rehabilitation and Physical Conditioning (pp 37-60).*
© 2014 SLACK Incorporated.

under certain conditions (such as arthritis), the patient is unable to tolerate or is limited with weight-bearing activity; therefore, aquatic therapy is ideal to encourage return to full weight-bearing function by practicing the movements in a partial weight-bearing environment.

Aquatic therapy is also advantageous for patients suffering from muscular injuries/fatigue who are unable to perform land-based exercise or when restricting muscle damage is indicated. Pantoja and coworkers assessed creatine kinase (CK) levels following resisted land-based and aquatic-based exercises and determined that a significant increase in CK was found 48 hours following exercise on land. Though significant differences were noted between land and water training, there was no significant difference pre- and postexercise in CK levels in individuals following aquatic exercise.[4]

Incorporating aquatic therapy into the rehabilitation/treatment has many advantages for the rehabilitation specialist who understands and applies the properties of water correctly. When developing a treatment plan, the rehabilitation specialist should incorporate the principles of tissue healing and determine appropriate exercise intensity and progression, all while considering the athlete's goals and treatment diagnosis. Depending upon the stage and aim of treatment, cardiovascular conditioning, range of motion (ROM) and stretching exercises, gait training, weight-bearing activities, and strengthening exercises can be incorporated and progressed to functional movement and sport-specific drills to allow the athlete to return to his or her desired level of function.

INDICATIONS FOR AQUATIC THERAPY

The incorporation of aquatic therapy into the rehabilitation program can profoundly affect the overall care of the patient. As always, consideration needs to be made of the contraindications to aquatic therapy. Once addressed, by employing water's buoyancy and resistant properties, as well as variable temperature control and hydrostatic pressure, the patient can achieve and attain improvements that may not be obtained with traditional land-based treatment at that same time postinjury. These improvements are achieved by allowing increased mobility, movement confidence, and activity tolerance with reduced pain[5,6] at a given stage of recovery.

Water provides surrounding support of the limb during movement, which allows for diminished complaints and guarding during movement activities. Aquatic therapy allows exercises to be performed when weight-bearing activities are permitted or recommended but not well tolerated by the patient, thus allowing closed kinetic chain (CKC) exercises to be initiated sooner than on land.[7,8] This allows earlier restoration of mobility and activity to impede the deleterious effects of inactivity associated with injury,

such as muscle atrophy, diminished joint mobility, and increased pain.[7,9,10]

There are 3 basic options when determining whether aquatic therapy is appropriate for a patient,[11] including wet-only therapy, dry-to-wet therapy, and wet-to-dry therapy. Wet-only therapy is utilized when patients have an inability to undertake or a decreased tolerance of land-based function and strengthening exercises or when they prefer aquatic exercises to land-based exercises. For patients who cannot bear their own weight (as in the case of those with diminished muscle capacity), the wet-only option enables them to increase cardiovascular activity and build muscle strength and endurance that can then be transferred into land-based function.

Dry-to-wet therapy is employed when land-based therapy exacerbates the patient's symptoms; the patient will therefore perform aquatic therapy until land-based exercises can be resumed without aggravating the patient's symptoms.

Wet-to-dry transition allows controlled progression of functional loading and is preferred when special consideration is needed for compressive loads, such as following certain surgical procedures or during rehabilitation of overuse injuries. In addition, aquatic therapy can be used in adjunct with land-based therapy as a means of alternating the patient's rehabilitation or training program.

IMMEDIATE POSTOPERATIVE WATERPROOFING FOR EARLY REHABILITATION

In a normal postsurgical wound that is free from signs of infections, it is important to create a barrier that will keep the wound completely dry during aquatic therapy. This can easily be accomplished with a bio-occlusive dressing. Multiple choices exist on the market and each clinician or facility will likely choose a favorite.

The most important part of obtaining good coverage and a constant dry environment for the wound is to ensure that the area around the incision/wound is clean and dry and is free of hair and oils or lotions. The next step is to position the extremity in the optimal position so that the wound remains protected throughout treatment. If covering an extensor surface, ensure that the extremity is in as much flexion as tolerated. Should you cover an extensor surface while it is in extension, the first significant flexion activity the patient does will likely disrupt the seal of the incision, causing the wound to become saturated. It is also vital that as you apply the dressing, you ensure that no wrinkles or creases are created that could channel moisture toward the wound. Practicing on extremities without open wounds to develop a proper technique is strongly encouraged.

When covering an immediate postoperative incision, it is also important to protect the sutures or closure devices. Some surgeons now use paper-like tape sometimes referred to as steri-strips. Regardless of whether the incision is stapled, sutured, or steri-stripped closed, you must protect the closure from the adhesive. Folding a piece of cotton gauze and running it along the incision will adequately protect it. Though the entire incision must be protected, if the piece of gauze that is utilized is too large, it could potentially compromise the dressing. Again, practice in applying dressings will aid in proper wound coverage and protection. The physical therapist should constantly be monitoring the dressing for any signs of loosening and remove the patient from the water should any sign of drainage appear. If the activity to be undertaken in the water involves or will create water turbulence, elasticated tubular support bandages over the dressing on a limb or joint can help prevent dressing edges from coming away from the skin, further ensuring dressing integrity. A bio-occlusive dressing is vital to eliminating the risk of infection. Maintaining proper pool chemistry will ensure it.

CASTS/BRACES

Protection of the patient is what makes aquatic therapy safe and successful. When a patient who is casted or braced enters the pool, special considerations and procedures should be taken to ensure that the cast stays dry and the extremity does not exceed any ROM limits. Multiple products exist that protect casts from moisture. Prior to application, it is important that the skin above or below the cast is clean and dry to ensure a proper seal.

The first treatment should be conservative and the patient and therapist must constantly assess the seal and fortitude of the protective sleeve. Once the protective sleeve has proven to be watertight, more aggressive exercises may be initiated.

Bracing is more about protecting the patient than it is about protecting the brace. Patients who have a diagnosis that limits ROM, such as immediate postoperative patellar tendon repair, ACL reconstruction, biceps tendon repair, or meniscus repair, should have a brace specifically designed and designated for pool use. The physical therapist will ensure that the brace is locked into the proper ROM prior to initiating treatment. This allows the patient to be confident in performing the exercises, knowing that he or she is not at risk of infection or injuring him- or herself. It also allows the physical therapist peace of mind that protocols will not be violated.

WARM-UP

A warm-up is essential prior to any physical treatment or exercise. A proper warm-up should be performed prior to activity and be gradual in intensity while preparing the body for the ensuing stretching, strengthening, or cardiovascular exercises to be performed. A warm-up performed in a therapeutic pool, especially one with an integrated underwater treadmill, is effective because the patient or athlete can engage in walking or jogging activities with the proper postural alignment and movement patterns versus a static pool floor. This allows the core body temperature to quickly rise, thus allowing increased circulation to the skeletal muscles faster.

A warm-up is performed for the purpose of increasing the temperature and circulation of the entire body and the muscular system. This is intended to reduce the incidence of musculoskeletal injuries, prepare the body for further strenuous activities during the ensuing workout, and diminish postworkout muscle soreness. The patient's specific warm-up will vary depending upon such variables as diagnosis, stage of recovery, available motion, and pain. The time required to perform a proper warm-up will vary depending upon each patient and the temperature of the water, with cooler water requiring a longer warm-up.

A total-body warm-up is encouraged prior to the initiation of activity with exercises performed by the upper extremity, determined by patient diagnosis and activity tolerance. If a pool with variable water depth is used, energy expenditure and perception of effort can be modified gradually to assist in the aquatic therapy goals, as shown by a University of Idaho case study authored by Dolny et al.[12] During the study, female participants walked on an underwater treadmill for a prescribed amount of time (six 5-min bouts) in a variety of different water depths; they also walked on a land-based treadmill for the same amount of time. During each walking bout, participants' heart rates, oxygen consumption, and carbon dioxide production were monitored and recorded. The results showed that minor changes in the depth of the pool water could significantly influence the cardiorespiratory variables and the subjects' perceptions of effort during aquatic exercise, especially as the water depth was adjusted by 20 cm.

LOWER BODY WARM-UP EXERCISES

Forward Walking

- Pool with traditional static floor: Patient is instructed to stand upright and flex the hip and knee on one side (Figure 4-1). Then while the patient leans slightly forward to create a forward momentum, the knee on this same leg is extended and the ankle is dorsiflexed and the patient lands on the unilateral heel. This is then repeated with the contralateral limb.
- Pool with underwater treadmill floor:
  - Walking on an underwater treadmill is easier to initiate than walking forward on a static pool floor,

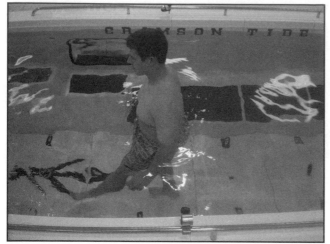

Figure 4-1. Forward walking.

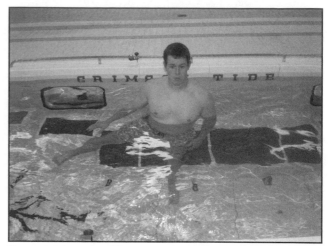

Figure 4-2. Lateral walking.

because on the treadmill you only need to overcome waters resistance to movement of the limbs, whereas in static pool walking, patients must overcome the resistance of the entire submerged body and thus a larger surface area.

○ Patients can walk at variable speeds, as indicated, with additional resistance being added through water jets, which can further load the forward propulsive movement pattern, if indicated.

○ Where available, adjustable water depth can also allow modification of relative weight-bearing status during performance of functional movements.

○ Patient's gait can be evaluated and corrected (if needed) via underwater video camera monitoring.

Backward Walking

• Pool with traditional static floor: Patient is instructed to stand upright and flex a unilateral hip and knee. The hip is extended posteriorly while the knee is extended and the ankle is plantarflexed, allowing the patient to land on the toes and gently roll onto the heel. This is then repeated with the contralateral limb.

• Pool with underwater treadmill floor:

○ Patient can walk backwards at variable speeds, as indicated. Additional resistance can be added using jets, if indicated.

○ Patient can use support bars on side of treadmill to increase stability.

○ Patient's toe/heel motion can be evaluated and corrected (if needed) via underwater video system monitoring.

Lateral Walking

• Pool with traditional static floor. Patient is instructed to stand upright with both legs straight (Figure 4-2).

The patient will make a lateral step by abducting the lead hip followed by bringing the foot to the pool floor, followed by adducting the opposite hip to the midline of the body and returning to the beginning standing position. This is then repeated in the opposite direction.

• Pool with underwater treadmill floor:

○ Patient can move laterally on the underwater treadmill (or treadmill floor). One may change speeds according to the patient's abilities. Additional resistance can be added using jets, if indicated.

○ Patient can use support bars on the side of the treadmill to increase stability during lateral movement.

○ Patient's lateral walking motions can be evaluated and corrected (if needed) via underwater video system monitoring.

Lateral Crossover Stepping

• Pool with traditional static floor: Patient is instructed to stand upright and adduct one leg anterior to the opposite leg and cross midline, allowing the foot to contact the pool floor, followed by abducting the opposite leg to return to the beginning standing position (Figure 4-3).

• Pool with underwater treadmill floor:

○ Patient can cross over during lateral walking on the underwater treadmill (or treadmill floor). Treadmill speeds can be changed according to the patient's abilities. Additional resistance can be added using jets, if indicated.

○ Patient can use support bars on the side of the treadmill to increase stability during crossover lateral movement.

○ Patient's lateral walking motions can be evaluated and corrected (if needed) via underwater video system monitoring.

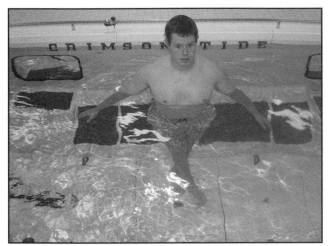

Figure 4-3. Lateral crossover stepping.

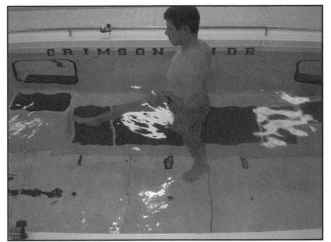

Figure 4-4. Straight-leg walking.

Straight-Leg Walking

- Pool with traditional static floor: Patient is instructed to stand upright and walk forward with both legs, keeping straight to fairly straight while both ankles are kept in a plantarflexed position (Figure 4-4).
- Pool with underwater treadmill floor:
  - Patient can use underwater treadmill to change straight-leg walking speeds. For increased resistance, resistance jets can be applied to change intensity.
  - Patient can make use of support bars on the side of the treadmill to increase stability during walking.
  - Patient's walking motions can be evaluated and corrected (if needed) via underwater video system monitoring.

Marching

- Pool with traditional static floor: Patient is instructed to stand upright and flex one hip and knee to 90 degrees and then bring the leg to the pool floor and flex the opposite hip and knee in a reciprocal marching manner. This is continued along with a comfortable arm swing throughout the marching.
- Pool with underwater treadmill floor:
  - Patient can use underwater treadmill to change speeds for marching. For increased resistance, resistance jets can be applied to change intensity.
  - Patient can make use of support bars on the side of the treadmill to increase stability during marching activity.

- Patient's hip and knee motions can be evaluated and corrected (if needed) via underwater video system monitoring.

Jogging

- Pool with traditional static floor: Patient is instructed to stand upright and perform a stationary jogging movement. This exercise should be performed at a comfortable speed and cadence for the patient with emphasis on correct movement pattern.
- Pool with underwater treadmill floor:
  - Patient can use underwater treadmill to change speeds as jogging becomes easier. For increased resistance, resistance jets can be applied to change intensities as indicated.
  - Patient can make use of support bars on the side of the embedded treadmill to increase stability.
  - Patient's walking motions can be evaluated and corrected (if needed) via underwater video system monitoring.

Deep Water Bicycle

- Patient is given a floatation device to allow for appropriate buoyancy and to maintain a vertical trunk (Figure 4-5). Patient performs reciprocating flexion and extension of both hips and knees to produce a vertical cyclic movement.
- Underwater treadmill pools with variable-depth floors can be utilized to safely change the pool floor level from shallow depths to depths up to 6 ft, depending on the patient's needs. This provides variety for deep water bicycle exercises.

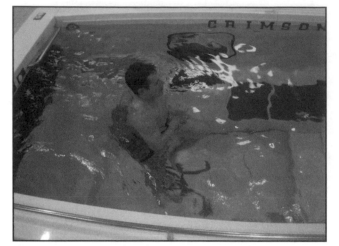

Figure 4-5. Deep water bicycle.

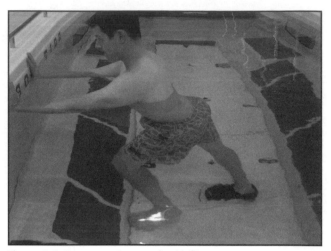

Figure 4-6. Gastrocnemius stretch with flipper.

FLEXIBILITY/RANGE OF MOTION/ MOBILITY EXERCISES

The therapeutic pool offers an ideal environment for ROM and flexibility activities due to the warmth of the water and also by allowing individuals who experience pain with weight-bearing activities to perform mobility exercises with diminished compressive loads. The patient is instructed to perform a low-intensity, long-duration (20 to 30 sec) stretch, because this has been shown to be the most effective in promoting lasting changes.[13] Below are some specific stretches that can be utilized for the lower extremity, which, depending upon the exercise, can be performed with or without the aid of buoyancy equipment. In the case of all stretching exercises, different loads can be maintained when performing aquatic therapy in a pool with a variable-depth floor.

Ankle and Foot Stretches

Gastrocnemius Stretch

The patient is instructed to face the pool wall and hold on to the edge of the pool or the support bars integrated into a pool with an embedded treadmill. With the involved knee maintained in an extended position and the heel remaining flat on the floor, the uninvolved limb is brought forward with the foot close to the pool wall, allowing the knee to flex to a comfortable position. The patient is instructed to extend the involved hip while maintaining the knee in an extended position and the heel remains in contact with the floor. This stretch can be enhanced by using a flipper to increase the length of the lever arm, which can make the stretch more comfortable and increase the effectiveness (Figure 4-6).

Soleus Stretch

The patient is instructed to face the pool wall and hold on to the edge of the pool or the support bars integrated into a pool with an embedded treadmill. With the involved knee maintained in an extended position and the heel remaining flat on the floor, the uninvolved limb is brought forward with the foot close to the pool wall or area where the support bars meet the floor, allowing the knee to flex to a comfortable position. The patient is instructed to extend the involved hip while maintaining heel contact with the floor while allowing the knee to flex until a comfortable stretch is obtained. This stretch can be enhanced by using a flipper to increase the length of the lever arm, which can make the stretch more comfortable and increase the effectiveness (Figure 4-7).

Plantar Fascia Stretch

The patient is instructed to hold on to the edge of the pool or the support bars integrated into a pool with an embedded treadmill with the chest against the pool wall or bars (Figure 4-8). The involved heel will be placed near the floor near the wall or lower part of the support bars while the toes are on the pool wall or against the support bars, with the knee maintained in slight flexion. The uninvolved leg is maintained in an extended position with the heel flat on the floor. The patient will push downward on the involved heel until a comfortable stretch is obtained.

Tibialis Anterior Stretch

The patient is instructed to stand erect while holding on to the pool wall or the support bars integrated into a pool with an embedded treadmill for support (Figure 4-9). The involved knee is flexed so that the dorsum of the foot and toes are on the pool floor. The patient is instructed to press the lower leg toward the floor, thereby creating a stretch on the anterior aspect of the lower leg. This stretch can be

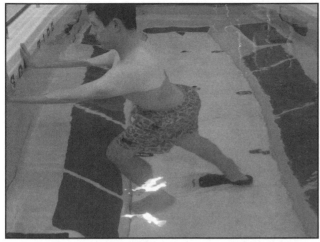

Figure 4-7. Soleus stretch with flipper.

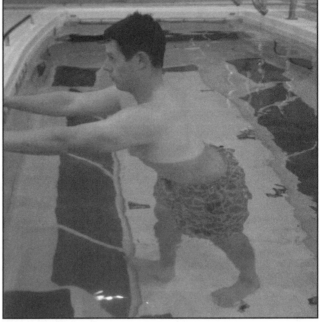

Figure 4-8. Plantar fascia stretch.

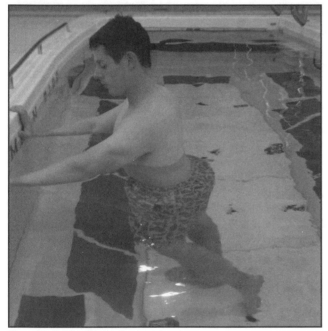

Figure 4-9. Tibialis anterior stretch.

enhanced by using a flipper to increase the length of the lever arm, which can make the stretch more comfortable and increase the effectiveness.

Knee Stretches

Quadriceps Stretch

The patient is instructed to hold on to the pool wall or the support bars integrated into a pool with an embedded treadmill for support. The involved knee is flexed and the patient holds on to the ankle while pulling the heel toward the buttocks until a comfortable stretch is achieved. The patient is instructed to maintain an erect trunk posture with the hip in an extended position.

Quadriceps Buoyancy-Assisted Stretch

A flotation device is placed around the ankle of the involved limb (Figure 4-10). The patient is instructed to hold on to the pool wall or the support bars integrated into a pool with an embedded treadmill for support and maintain the trunk in an upright position with trunk, hips, and knees in a vertical alignment. The knee is then allowed to flex with the assistance of the flotation device to achieve a stretch on the quadriceps musculature.

Hamstring Stretch

The patient is instructed to place the involved foot on the pool ladder at a comfortable height and maintain ankle dorsiflexion. The uninvolved foot is placed at a comfortable distance behind the patient. The patient is instructed to maintain an erect trunk and bend forward at the hips until a comfortable stretch is achieved in the hamstring.

Hamstring Buoyancy-Assisted Stretch

A flotation device is placed around the ankle of the involved limb (Figure 4-11). The patient is instructed to hold on to the pool wall or the support bars integrated into a pool with an embedded treadmill for support and maintain the trunk in an upright position with trunk, hips, and knees in a vertical alignment. The hip is then allowed to extend with the assistance of the flotation device to achieve a stretch on the hamstring musculature.

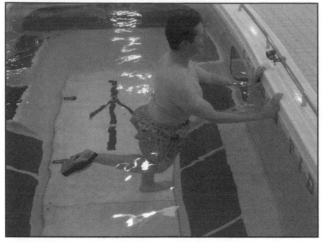

Figure 4-10. Quadriceps buoyancy-assisted stretch.

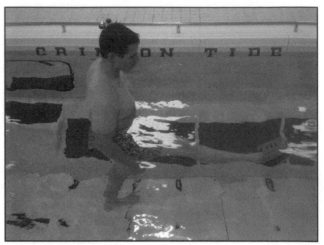

Figure 4-11. Hamstring buoyancy-assisted stretch.

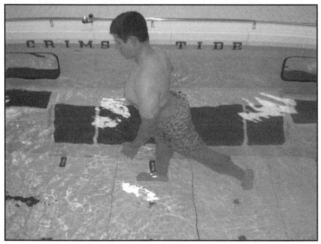

Figure 4-12. Hip flexor stretch.

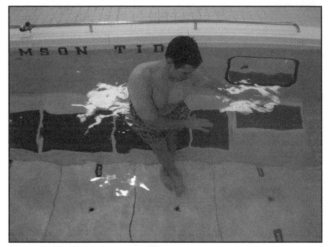

Figure 4-13. Hip abductor stretch.

Hip Stretches

Hip Flexor Stretch

The patient is instructed to step forward with the non-involved leg with the knee maintained in a flexed position; the involved leg is positioned behind the patient with the knee in extension (Figure 4-12). The patient is instructed to maintain an erect trunk and push the involved hip forward until a stretch is achieved in the hip flexors. In a pool with an integrated treadmill, the embedded support bars can help with support. Additionally, resistance jets can be utilized to provide increased intensity.

Hip Abductor Stretch

The patient is instructed to stand with the trunk erect and cross the involved leg in front of the other leg (Figure 4-13). The patient is then instructed to lean to the uninvolved side without bending forward at the waist, while adducting the involved hip until a comfortable stretch is achieved in the hip abductors. In a pool with an underwater treadmill, the integrated support bars can help with stability. Additionally, resistance jets can be utilized to provide increased intensity.

An alternate patient position for stretching the hip abductors and iliotibial band can be performed using a step or ladder. The patient is instructed to place the foot of the involved leg on to a comfortable step of the ladder and, while maintaining a neutral trunk, slightly horizontally adduct the leg across the midline. The patient is then instructed to rotate the hip internally until a comfortable stretch is achieved in the hip abductors.

Hip Adductor Stretch

The patient is instructed to stand with the trunk erect with the feet facing forward and placed more than shoulder width apart (Figure 4-14). The patient is then instructed to lean to the opposite side of the involved leg while the trunk is maintained in a neutral position until a comfortable stretch is achieved in the hip adductors. This stretch can be modified by placing the involved foot onto a step or the ladder to increase the amount of hip adduction attained.

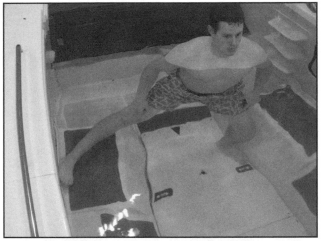

Figure 4-14. Hip adductor stretch.

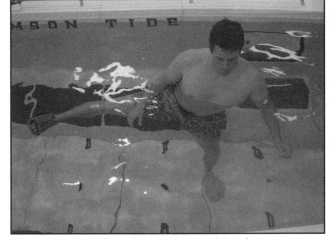

Figure 4-15. Hip adductor buoyancy-assisted stretch.

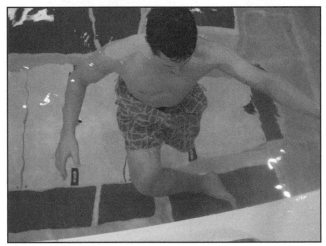

Figure 4-16. Hip piriformis stretch.

Hip Adductor Buoyancy-Assisted Stretch

A flotation device is placed around the ankle of the involved limb (Figure 4-15). The patient is instructed to hold on to the pool wall or the support bars integrated into a pool with an embedded treadmill for support and maintain the trunk in an upright position with trunk, hips, and knees in a vertical alignment. The hip is then allowed to abduct with the assistance of the flotation device to achieve a stretch on the adductor musculature.

Hip Piriformis Stretch

The patient is instructed to maintain the trunk in an erect, neutral position and position the involved leg in a figure-4 position onto a step or railing (Figure 4-16). The patient is then instructed to squat and flex the trunk until a comfortable stretch is achieved. The patient can modify the intensity of the stretch by altering the amount of trunk flexion, adjusting the amount of horizontal hip abduction and external rotation, and altering the amount of contralateral knee flexion by squatting with the contralateral (stance) leg.

DYNAMIC FLEXIBILITY AND RANGE OF MOTION EXERCISES

Dynamic ROM activities are designed to not only improve muscular flexibility but to increase joint mobility and improve coordination. These activities can be performed in deep water (the level of which can be efficiently changed in a pool with a variable-depth, adjustable floor) to allow activities in a nonweight-bearing fashion; these exercises include deep water bicycling, frog legs, bent-knee hip rotations, cross-country skiing, and jumping jacks. These exercises vary in movements, muscle activity, and knee motion; the rehabilitation specialist should use discretion when prescribing these activities; for example, the patient may only perform cross-country skiing and jumping jacks when desiring to limit the amount of knee flexion. Examples of dynamic flexibility exercises performed in neck-deep or shallow water include jumping jacks, cross-country skiing, walking lunges, and lateral lunges, where the stride is increased to focus on increased mobility of the hip, knee, and ankle joints.

STRENGTHENING EXERCISES

Isometric Exercises

Isometric exercises are indicated when joint movement is contraindicated or cannot be performed due to pain with active motion. In addition, electromyographic (EMG) activity has been shown to be decreased when performing maximal and submaximal isometric contractions in the water compared to on dry land.[14] This could benefit an individual who is having pain or apprehension with exercises or activities. Isometric exercises can be performed using the pool wall or the support bars integrated into a pool with an embedded treadmill as a resistive force as in Figure 4-17.

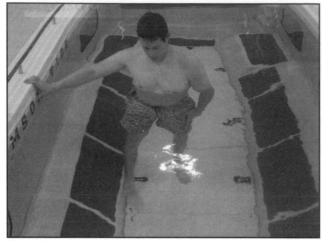

Figure 4-17. Hip isometric abduction on the pool wall.

Isometric exercises can also be performed in a single-leg stance in turbulent water, which is made easier with the addition of hydraulic resistance jets (found in technologically advanced pools with embedded underwater treadmill systems). The direction of the turbulence can be changed to modify the musculature emphasized for stabilization. In addition, this turbulence can be created through patient arm motion, through practitioner movements, or from pool resistance jets or turbines (Figure 4-18).

Isotonic Exercises

Isotonic strengthening exercises can be performed either in an open kinetic chain (OKC) or CKC manner. Incorporating both forms of exercise into the rehabilitation program is generally beneficial, but the rehabilitation specialist should determine which form of exercises should be performed based on tolerance, diagnosis, and treatment goals. Water provides an excellent medium for performing isotonic strengthening exercises. Though the principles of exercise and strength training are similar for programs performed on dry land and in the water, the physiologic responses are not necessarily the same. Unlike traditional strengthening equipment, which offers resistance in only one plane of motion, resistance exercises performed in an aquatic environment provide resistance in all directions of movement. The resistance of the exercise can be modified by the speed of movement, the use of resistive equipment, altering the water turbulence via hydraulically driven resistance jets, altering the depth of the pool, and adjusting the lever arm.

Open Kinetic Chain Exercises

Pöyhönen and coworkers reported on a single-repetition knee extension/flexion movement and a repeated (6 to 8 repetitions) extension/flexion movement during OKC knee extension performed in water while barefoot.[15] It was noted that during single-repetition knee extension testing

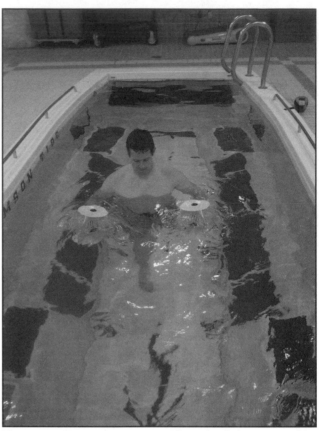

Figure 4-18. Hip isometric stance with pool turbulence created by upper extremity movement.

the highest amount of quadriceps activity was observed between 110 and 70 degrees, and the EMG activity of the antagonist hamstrings was low during the movement. They reported a mean peak angular velocity of 470 degrees/sec in men and 480 degrees/sec in women during extension and 470 degrees/sec in men and 375 degrees/sec in women during flexion. During the repeated extension/flexion testing, the quadriceps EMG peaked at 100 degrees in both groups and activity decreased from an angle of 75 degrees to full extension, whereas the antagonistic hamstring EMGs during knee extension started to increase at 80 degrees in men and 70 degrees in women.[15] During active knee flexion, the hamstring activity declined from 40 to 115 degrees, whereas the quadriceps (antagonist) increased from 40 to 115 degrees, and during repeated extension/flexion movements the antagonistic hamstring EMG started to increase at 80 degrees during active knee extension with a corresponding decrease in quadriceps activity throughout the remaining arc of motion.[15] Therefore, based on these findings and depending on the aim and goal of the exercise activity, the rehabilitation specialist can alter the amount of antagonistic muscle activity by having the patient perform single-repetition exercises to isolate agonist muscle activity or perform repeated movements to increase the activity of the antagonistic muscles.

OKC exercises can use either viscosity or buoyancy to provide the necessary resistance during strengthening

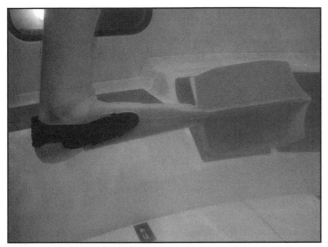

Figure 4-19. Ankle plantarflexion/dorsiflexion utilizing fin for added resistance.

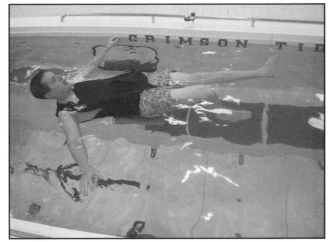

Figure 4-20. Supine buoyancy-resisted knee flexion.

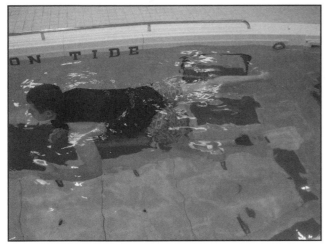

Figure 4-21. Prone knee extension with flipper.

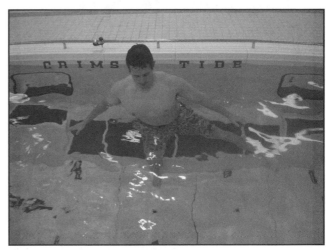

Figure 4-22. Triplanar hip strengthening.

exercises. OKC exercises for the ankle/foot utilizing the viscous properties of water can be accomplished using a flipper or fin (Figure 4-19). In this example, the exercise equipment provides an increased lever arm requiring increased torque production. A buoyant strap or footwear device allows the user to perform resisted exercises with buoyancy providing the resistance. OKC exercises can also be performed in a variety of ways. Figure 4-20 demonstrates knee flexion performed while floating supine utilizing buoyancy to provide the necessary resistance, and Figure 4-21 demonstrates resisted knee extension utilizing fins while in a prone position. Figure 4-22 displays the ability to perform triplanar movements during aquatic therapy as the patient performs a diagonal hip-strengthening exercise. The practitioner can also utilize resistive bands to provide the necessary resistance during strengthening exercises as demonstrated in Figure 4-23 as the patient performs hip extension strengthening exercises. Commercial equipment can allow for resisted movements; for example, the Hydro-Boot (Hydro-Tone Fitness Systems, Inc, Yorba Linda, CA;

Figure 4-24), which can be utilized to increase the resistance as much as 4-fold during movement.[16,17]

Pöyhönen and coworkers studied the relationship of EMG activity and velocity during knee extension/flexion in men and women performing isokinetics at 180 degrees/sec and in the water both barefoot and while wearing a Hydro-Boot with maximum effort.[18] They reported that in the barefoot condition, men produced higher velocities than women during extension (364 ± 120 degrees/sec versus 302 ± 110 degrees/sec) and flexion (326 ± 30 degrees/sec versus 296 ± 33 degrees/sec). With the Hydro-Boot, the means of angular velocity in men was higher than women during extension (210 ± 73 degrees/sec versus 193 ± 72 degrees/sec), whereas there was no difference in the mean velocity in flexion (174 ± 54 degrees/sec versus 168 ± 62 degrees/sec). During knee extension the subjects reached the peak drag at a knee flexion angle of 70 degrees in the barefoot condition and 60 degrees with the Hydro-Boot. In addition, the peak drag values in extension were greater with the Hydro-Boot (209 ± 46 N in men,

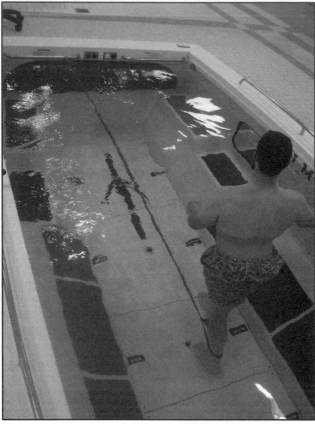

Figure 4-23. Hip extension strengthening using elastic resistance.

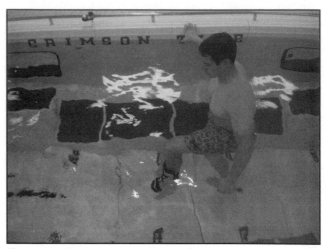

Figure 4-24. Knee extension using a Hydro-Boot.

145 ± 30 N in women) compared to the barefoot condition (89 ± 43 N in men, 45 ± 15 N in women). This produced a percentage maximum voluntary contraction (MVC) of 104 ± 18 with the Hydro-Boot and 124 ± 18 while barefoot. During flexion, the peak drag values with the Hydro-Boot were 176 ± 50 N in men and 137 ± 26 N in women, and the peak drag values when barefoot were 98 ± 30 N in men and 55 ± 13 N in women, with peak drag occurring at 40 degrees, producing a percentage MVC with the Hydro-Boot of 120 ± 20 for men and 128 ± 21 for women. Based on these studies.[14,15,18] OKC activities may be performed with diminished stress placed upon the ACL as a result of the reduced activity of the quadriceps, with a simultaneous increased activation of the hamstrings during the last 30 to 40 degrees of knee extension, which prevents excessive anterior shear forces, thereby reducing ACL strain.

Closed Kinetic Chain Exercises

CKC exercises performed in the water utilize buoyancy to reduce relative weight-bearing status and thus load. This may allow patients to perform exercises traditionally accepted as being of benefit to rehab progression earlier and more comfortably than they could have been performed pain and irritation free on land. In pools with variable height adjustment, CKC exercises can be safely progressed toward full weight-bearing load, mimicking the results of similar land-based exercises without the same full weight-bearing-related stress. Some examples of CKC exercises that can be performed are step-ups (Figure 4-25), double- (Figure 4-26) and single-leg squats (Figure 4-27), lunge squats (Figure 4-28), and calf raises. In fact, most exercises that can be performed full weight bearing can be adapted to the water environment, normally at an earlier stage in a rehabilitation program due the various qualities of water. CKC exercises can be performed in a variety of ways as well, to allow for patient comfort as well as to adjust the intensity of the exercise. For example, variations in the squat exercise

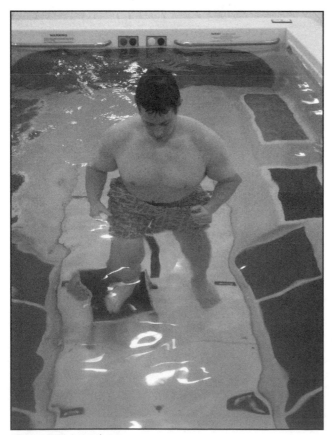

Figure 4-25. Lateral step-up.

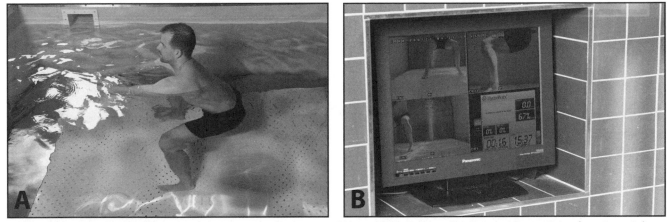

Figure 4-26. (A) Double-leg squats. (B) Underwater video assessment of hip and knee position. (Reprinted with permission from Jason Palmer, BHMS (Ed) Hons, BPhty, MCSP.)

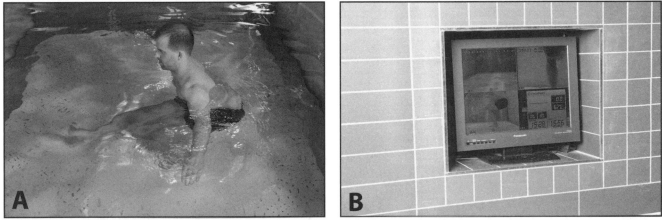

Figure 4-27. (A) Single-leg squats. (B) Underwater analysis of knee alignment. (Reprinted with permission from Jason Palmer, BHMS (Ed) Hons, BPhty, MCSP.)

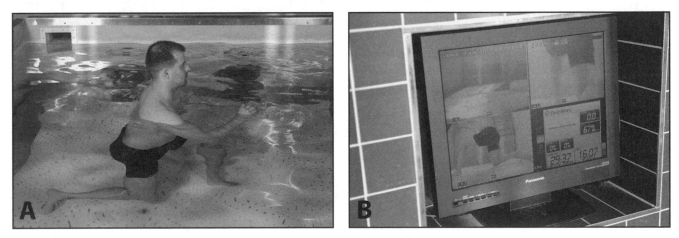

Figure 4-28. (A) Forward lunge. (B) Assessment of lunge stride and alignment using underwater video. (Reprinted with permission from Jason Palmer, BHMS (Ed) Hons, BPhty, MCSP.)

include deep water squats, shallow water squats, supine buoyancy-supported squats (Figure 4-29), and squatting with resistive equipment (Figure 4-30).

Buoyancy equipment can be used to provide the needed resistance during CKC exercises. The patient can place a noodle under the involved foot and from a starting position of hip and knee flexion, the patient is instructed to extend the hip and knee and perform a buoyancy-resisted single-leg press movement (Figure 4-31). The use of a buoyancy device requires increased coordination and eccentric control. Incorporating arm movements during activities such as walking drills or lunges can increase the resistance of

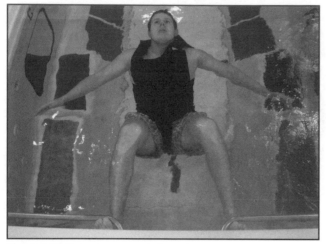

Figure 4-29. Buoyancy-supported squats.

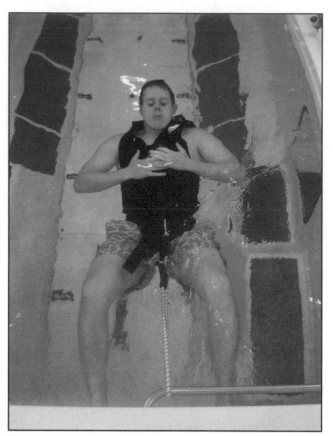

Figure 4-30. Buoyancy-supported resisted squat.

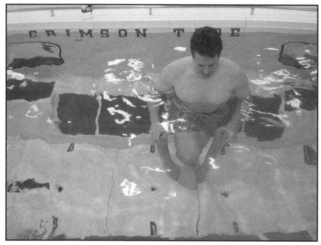

Figure 4-31. Buoyancy-resisted single leg press.

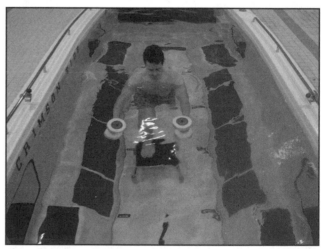

Figure 4-32. Forward lunge onto step using buoyant dumbbells for trunk stabilization.

the exercise and allow for total body training (Figure 4-32). To further augment arm movements, the patient can wear aqua gloves or perform upper extremity push–pull movements with buoyant dumbbells (Figure 4-33). Exercise intensity can also be increased by decreasing the rest intervals and increasing the speed of movement.

PROPRIOCEPTIVE TRAINING

Proprioceptive and balance training drills in both static and dynamic postures are essential components to a comprehensive rehabilitation program. The pool, particularly when fitted with an integrated underwater treadmill, moveable floor, and resistance jets, provides an excellent medium for proprioceptive training in individuals who experience difficulty performing weight-bearing activities on dry land due to lower extremity weakness or pain during stance or when full weight bearing is contraindicated.

Performing balance training in the water also allows the patient to exercise without the fear of falling, even

when walking briskly on an underwater treadmill. This is because the viscous properties of the water and the reduction of the effects of gravity through water's buoyancy reduce the speed of falling when balance is lost, giving the patient greater time for postural corrections. Balance, proprioception, and postural control are influenced by joint and tissue proprioceptors, visual cues, and vestibular feedback. Therefore, the difficulty of the exercise can be altered by challenging these systems; for example, by

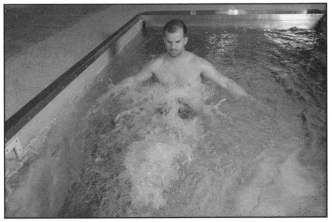

Figure 4-34. Single leg balance in turbulent water. (Reprinted with permission from Jason Palmer, BHMS (Ed) Hons, BPhty, MCSP.)

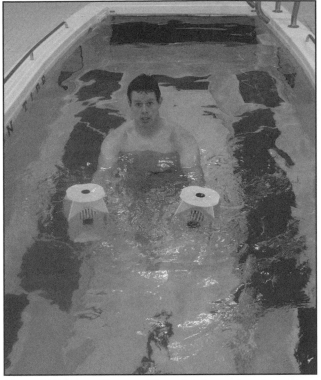

Figure 4-33. Forward lunges while performing push–pull movement with Hydro-Bells (Hydro-Tone Fitness Systems, Inc).

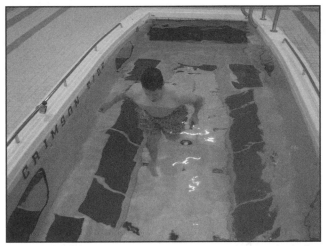

Figure 4-36. Single-leg stance while depressing a buoyant barbell to increase trunk sway.

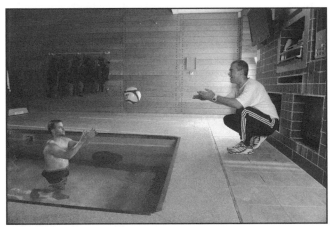

Figure 4-35. Single leg balance with ball toss. (Reprinted with permission from Jason Palmer, BHMS (Ed) Hons, BPhty, MCSP.)

adding turbulence to the water through resistance jets, using eyes open and closed drills (Figure 4-34), using visual distraction activities such as balancing while also focusing on other objects/tasks such as catching a ball (Figure 4-35) or looking at objects around the environment, performing a single-leg stance while pushing a buoyant barbell down with the upper extremity (Figure 4-36), as well as having the patient perform balance activity while standing on various buoyant devices such as a wafer, noodle, or buoyant barbell (Figure 4-37) in open- or closed-chain drills. In addition, the patient can perform squats while standing on a buoyant exercise device such as a buoyant barbell or a floating wedge (Figure 4-38) and can be challenged with

perturbations through water currents created by either water jets or manual turbulence created by the therapist.

FUNCTIONAL TRAINING

The key to a successful rehabilitation outcome is the ability of the patient to return to his or her desired functional level. Early restoration of functional movement patterns is considered essential in an accelerated rehab process, and water-based therapy can have a significant influence on achieving these goals.

For some patients, independent walking around the shopping center once a week may be the goal, whereas for others the dynamic movement demands of an elite sport may be the target. Regardless of any patient's functional target, water and the current water-based technologies such as underwater treadmills offer an environment that can be adapted to meet the needs of even the most demanding patients.

Running, for example, is one of the most basic functional activities and is integral to many sporting and active leisure

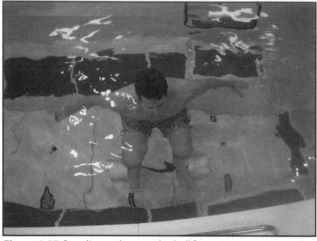

Figure 4-37. Standing on buoyant barbell for proprioception training.

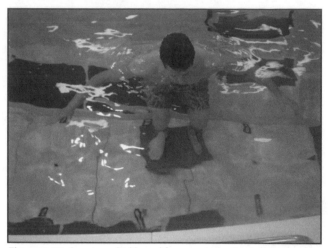

Figure 4-38. Squats on kickboard for proprioception training.

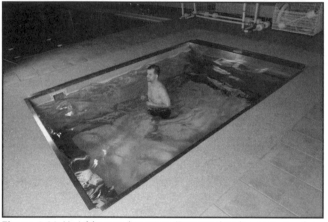

Figure 4-39. Variable speed jogging. (Reprinted with permission from Jason Palmer, BHMS (Ed) Hons, BPhty, MCSP.)

pursuits. Water running can be introduced very early in many rehab programs through complete nonweight-bearing activities; that is, deep water running sessions and then progressed through to sessions at 50% weight bearing. These sessions can be undertaken on static floor pools or those with underwater treadmills. Aquatic treadmill exercise is superior for progression of this type of work because more normal movement patterns and greater functional speeds can be achieved in running because the patient does not need to overcome the drag forces of moving the entire submerged body through the water as is required in static pool sessions; that is, the moving floor permits faster limb speeds. Normally water depth needs only be reduced to 50% weight-bearing depth in any progression because the normal functional movement of the limbs is initiated from the core or trunk, but once the trunk is no longer at least partly in the water, it does not experience the increased resistant forces as the legs and therefore movement patterns alter. With increased movement speeds, movements become labored as the patient tries to move the limbs through water and consequently the nature of the movement becomes less functional. Fortunately, however, experience has shown us

that once a patient can perform good quality work at this 50% weight-bearing level, he or she is ready to begin the transition to full weight-bearing activity. A logical progression could, for example, be an athlete progressing from running at 4 to 5 mph on the underwater treadmill with good form and movement quality to an introduction to jogging at slower speeds on land (100% weight bearing). Thus, functional movement intensity (running speed) is reduced with the transition but the weight-bearing load is increased through moving from 50% to 100% weight bearing and so progression does occur.

There are few functional movement patterns, from those of basic activities of daily living through to those of elite sport, that cannot be performed and progressed (often earlier than on land) in the water, from basic sit-to-stand movements, through linear walking and running patterns at variable speeds (Figure 4-39) and multidirection movements (Figure 4-40). The patient can, for example, perform such activities as lateral cone walking drills (Figure 4-41) to dynamic power-based jump-and-land activities (Figure 4-42); all that is required to include these in water-based rehabilitation is an understanding of the basic building blocks of the desired movement, the ability to design a progressively overloaded program that takes a patient safely from the most basic level of the activity to the final outcome, and a little imagination. Even the fittest and strongest of athletes can be challenged in the water environment, particularly when the therapist has at his or her disposal the ability to use and adjust environmental parameters such as water depth, treadmill speed, visual feedback and movement resistance (ie, use of jet water currents; Figure 4-43).

Functional activities should be incorporated throughout the training program as they are tolerated and as indicated or determined by healing constraints as well as sport/activity demands. Where possible, include specific sport-based movement patterns and skills for patient motivation and enjoyment, using familiar games as part of the program (Figure 4-44). It is important in the planning process,

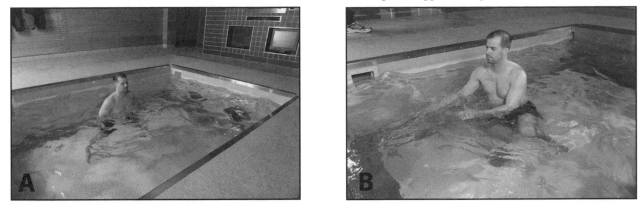

Figure 4-40. (A) Core stabilization with multidirectional hip movements. (B) Synchronizing hip and trunk movements during triplanar hip motions. (Reprinted with permission from Jason Palmer, BHMS (Ed) Hons, BPhty, MCSP.)

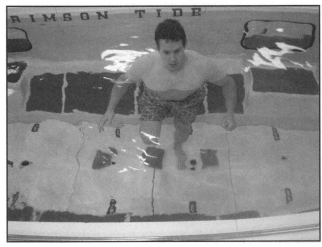

Figure 4-41. Lateral cone walking drills

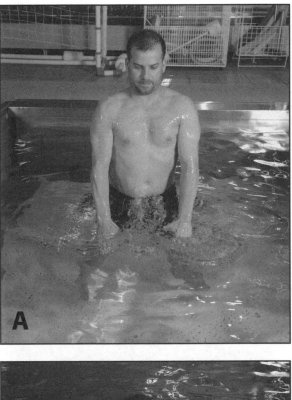

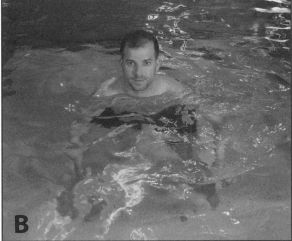

Figure 4-42. (A) Vertical jumping. (B) Landing drills with instruction to land softly with hips and knees slightly flexed. (Reprinted with permission from Jason Palmer, BHMS (Ed) Hons, BPhty, MCSP.)

however, that the therapist consider how the water will challenge the patient and his or her pathology. For example, because of the viscosity of the water, careful consideration needs to be given to any possible stresses/strains, as in performing lateral movements with a patient diagnosed with a medial collateral ligament strain due to the valgus stress that may occur during hip adduction.

For sporting activities that require impact, the pool can be utilized to introduce explosive exercises with reduced impact on the lower extremity, such as repetitive jumps. The athlete is encouraged to learn appropriate landing techniques, including landing with knees bent and avoiding excessive knee valgus. The athlete begins with jumping and landing drills involving both legs and progresses to single-leg activities. The patient can perform jump landing from steps of varying height, tethered wall push-offs (Figure 4-45), and barbell jump-overs (Figure 4-46). The trainer can also utilize the underwater treadmill's hydraulic jets to add resistance via water turbulence and use an underwater video camera to monitor the patient's progress (and make necessary adjustments).

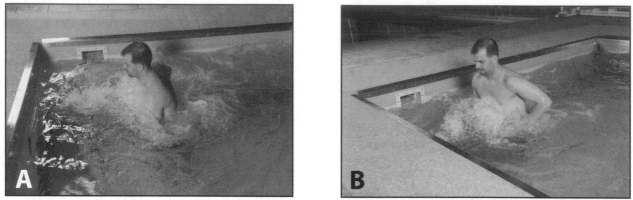

Figure 4-43. Jet speed can be adjusted to allow for both (A) jogging and (B) sprinting. (Reprinted with permission from Jason Palmer, BHMS (Ed) Hons, BPhty, MCSP.)

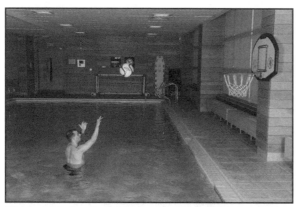

Figure 4-44. Sporting activities provide motivation and incorporate functional movement patterns. (Reprinted with permission from Jason Palmer, BHMS (Ed) Hons, BPhty, MCSP.)

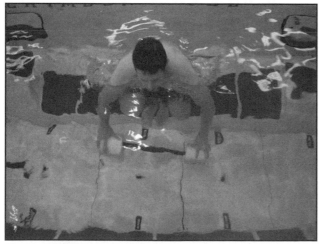

Figure 4-46. Buoyancy barbell jump-overs.

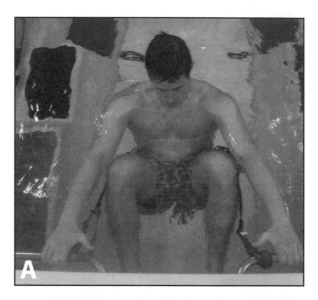

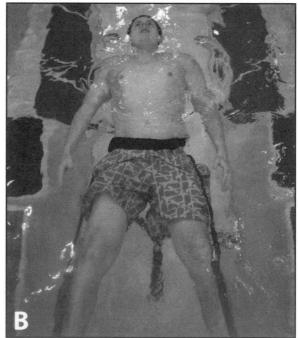

Figures 4-45. (A) Tethered wall push-offs (starting position). (B) Tethered wall push-offs (ending position).

PLYOMETRIC TRAINING

Plyometric and jumping activities are an essential part of the return to training/playing part of rehabilitation, which uses dynamic movements to stimulate the "power" component of muscle/tendon function and joint coordination. Water offers a fantastic environment to develop this

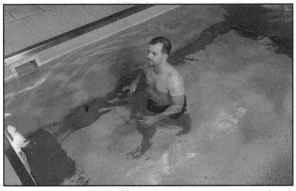

Figure 4-47. Jogging in chest deep water to minimize lower extremity joint reaction forces. (Reprinted with permission from Jason Palmer, BHMS (Ed) Hons, BPhty, MCSP.)

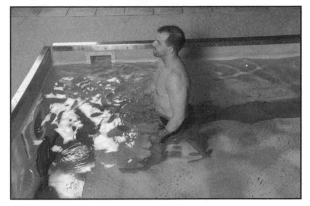

Figure 4-48. Jogging in waist deep water to increase lower extremity joint reaction forces. (Reprinted with permission from Jason Palmer, BHMS (Ed) Hons, BPhty, MCSP.)

dynamic movement and through its various qualities allows a progressively overloaded program to be delivered with a greater degree of safety than that of a land-only program. Plyometrics in the pool have been shown to have a significantly greater amount of concentric force production and increased rate of force development while incurring lower impact forces compared to dry-land jumping[19] and thus less eccentric loading. Due to the diminished impact forces produced during aquatic therapy and the decreased muscle damage incurred with aquatic therapy compared to land-based exercises, aquatic plyometric exercises can effectively be included as part of any training and rehabilitation program for lower extremities.[4] Normally, aquatic plyometrics can be implemented earlier than land-based plyometric activities, because water's buoyancy reduces the impact load relative to full weight bearing and is thus safer and more comfortable. Adjustable water depth, for example, can be used to progress function from minimal weight-bearing environments of approximately 30% weight bearing (water approximately at chest depth; Figure 4-47) to 50% weight-bearing environments where the water is approximately at waist level (Figure 4-48). As with other dynamic activities such as running, once water depth reaches waist level, any further reduction in depth can have an impact on performance.

Almost any functional movement can be adapted to the water, broken down into smaller stages, and then rebuilt to the point where the activity can be reintroduced on land. For example, if the goal is to be able to jump off one leg following knee surgery, a progression would be safe walking progressing to jogging in deep water moving toward more shallow water. At the same time, basic functional strength exercises such as bilateral squat movements progress to single-leg movements, which similarly progress from deeper to shallow water. Then bilateral jumps can be introduced and progress as above until the athlete is able to perform a single-leg jump and land on the same leg with quality in waist-deep water. The key is to design a program that at no stage takes too large a step or progression that could undermine a patient's performance quality or confidence. Plyometric aquatic training has been shown to improve vertical jumping.[20] A vertical jump is an explosive movement of the entire body that involves contributions of the upper extremity, torso, and lower extremity. A vertical jump that incorporates upper extremity movement allows an individual to jump higher as a result of influencing the stretch shortening cycle by slowing down the muscular contraction of the lower extremity and therefore generates greater force production and a greater angular knee extension velocity (increased by 28%); upper extremity movement also produces a 72% increase in trunk velocity and raises the body's center of gravity by 54%.[21-25] Therefore, we utilize various water depths during our plyometric training with shallow water to isolate lower extremity (Figures 4-49 and 4-50) or deep water to incorporate upper extremity training during plyometric activity (Figure 4-51).

Underwater Treadmill Running at 10% to 25% Weight-Bearing Status

Underwater treadmill running at neck- to chest-deep water depth is a biomechanically preferred method to maintain or even improve an athlete's conditioning status during the rehabilitation process. It provides a nearly pain-free and impact-free alternative to land conditioning. It also can be an experience where the athlete's condition progresses by gradually increasing the treadmill speed (for example, from 4 to 8 mph) and the frontal jet resistance. The combination of increasing treadmill speed and increasing jet resistance will help get the athlete reconditioned and "game ready" before he or she returns to land activities.

According to Alberto Salazar,[12] the Olympic distance coach for Mo Farah and Galen Rupp of the Nike Oregon Project, there are 4 key areas that must be considered when

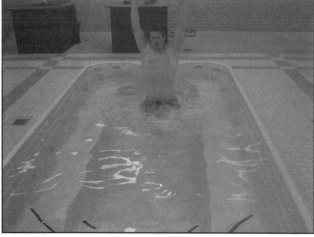

Figure 4-49. Shallow water vertical jump.

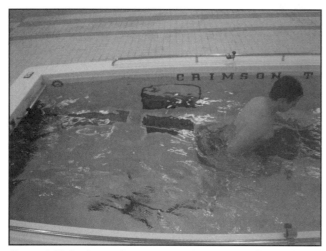

Figure 4-51. Stationary deep water running using a tether cord.

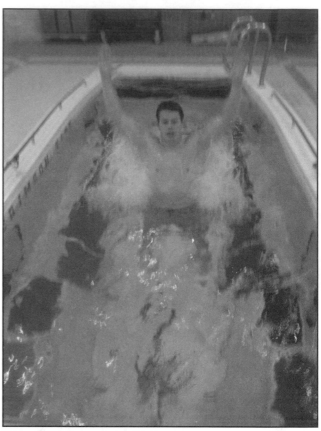

Figure 4-50. Deep water vertical jump.

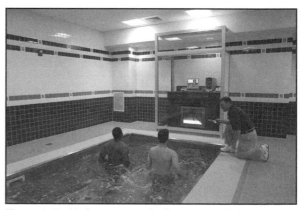

Figure 4-52. Underwater treadmill running with biomechanical video feedback on form. (Reprinted with permission from HydroWorx.)

adding underwater treadmill running to an athlete's rehabilitation or conditioning program:

1. Posture: The way one holds one's body in water while running against the resistance or viscosity of the water (which is much stronger than air) tends to become sloppy and an exaggerated forward lean results if posture is not consistently considered. A good rule of thumb for low to moderate running intensities is to ensure that the body follows a plumb line. That is, if a line were drawn from the ear to the hip to the ankle (when the athlete is in profile), the line would be straight. If the body is bent forward, adjustments should be made immediately. Use an underwater video system to ensure correct posture so that physical corrections can be seen and made by both the athlete and the therapist or athletic trainer. As the intensity progresses to higher levels, there will be a natural slight forward incline to the running style, which is normal.

2. Gait and stride length: As with posture, an athlete's gait in water is different than on land. Legs are being propelled through a relatively dense material (when compared to air), so the gait must be monitored and

modified when necessary (Figure 4-52). For most athletes, the gait used is specific to that person and should be applied in the water on an underwater treadmill as well. There is no "one way" to run on an underwater treadmill, and it is important to monitor the athlete's form and coach him or her to run in his or her correct biomechanical movement patterns. Underwater video monitoring is effective for helping the athlete adapt his or her form to his or her true land-based running form.

3. Foot strike: The athlete must be prepared to use the proper foot strike techniques when running on an underwater treadmill at chest-deep levels or greater.

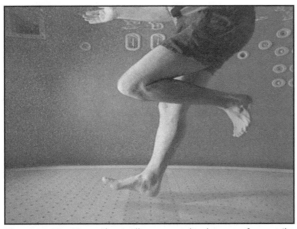

Figure 4-53. Biomechanically correct heel-to-toe foot strike on underwater treadmill. (Reprinted with permission from HydroWorx.)

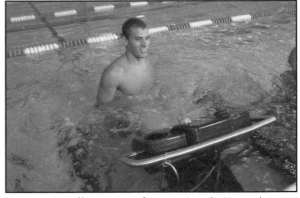

Figure 4-54. Efficient use of arm swing during underwater treadmill running. (Reprinted with permission from HydroWorx.)

Like gait patterns, foot strikes vary greatly. Each type of foot strike (heel-to-toe or balls-of-feet running) will produce different cardiovascular responses and the athlete should be counseled to run in correct biomechanical form to his land foot striking patterns (Figure 4-53). Again, underwater video is helpful in this process.

4. Arm swing: Arms play an important role while running on land as well as underwater. On land, they are used to help propel the body; in an aquatic environment, they can actually slow a runner's progression if he or she is positioned in a sloppy manner. The arms should be slashing thru the water as they would on land, and this takes concentration and the splashing created by the arms and hands should be minimal (Figure 4-54). The arms should be moving efficiently back and forth, and underwater video monitoring can be used to correct the athlete's arm movements when necessary.

DEEP WATER RUNNING

Deep water running (DWR) can serve as an effective form of cardiovascular conditioning and as an impact-free workout (see Figure 4-44). DWR is performed with a flotation device (vest or belt) to allow for stabilization and ensure that the head is above water. The patient can run in a stationary position by using a tether cord or run across the pool. Because the patient is running in deep water, there is no contact with the bottom of the pool; therefore, weight bearing forces are eliminated and running form should closely mirror that of dry-land running. An underwater video camera with a monitor can also help the trainer ensure the patient is maintaining safe form.

The following are general guidelines used when instructing an individual in proper form during DWR[26,27]:

- The water should be at shoulder level with the mouth comfortably out of the water and the head held in a neutral position with a tilt.

- The trunk should be maintained in a neutral position in a slightly forward tilted position.

- The arm motion should be identical to that used during land running; the elbows should be bent and the arm swing should primarily occur at the shoulder, with the hands reaching to just below the waterline approximately 8 to 12 in from the chest during flexion and just below the hip during extension.

- Hip flexion should reach 60 to 80 degrees during stride with the leg extending at the knee from the flexed position. As maximum hip flexion is reached, the opposite leg should reach a perpendicular position. The hip and knee should be extended together and achieve full knee extension and neutral hip flexion (0 degrees) in unison. Then as the hip goes into hyperextension, the knee should be brought into flexion and this cycle is then repeated.

- The ankle should be dorsiflexed when the hip is in neutral and the knee should be extended and plantarflexed as the hip is hyperextended and the knee is flexed. The ankle should return to a dorsiflexed position as the hip is flexed and knee is extended.

When prescribing water running time should be used for training purposes. Deep water running can be monitored and prescribed based upon heart rate, time, cadence, and rating of perceived exertion. Sprinters may run for intervals of 10 to 90 sec, distance runners 5 to 10 min, and marathoners 2 to 4 hours. The Brennan Scale was designed for deep water running and can be used to determine and monitor exertion rate. This scale ranges from 1 to 5 with 1 described as a light jog, 2 as long run, 3 as somewhat hard, 4 as a hard long sprint, and 5 as very hard (eg, a 100- to 200-m sprint.) Cadence, defined as the number of times the right leg moves through a complete gait cycle each minute, is another means of monitoring exercise intensity.[27] Wilder et al showed a high correlation between cadence and heart

Table 4-1.

	Deep Water Cadence to Land Equivalent Running Chart	
RPE	**Aqua Running (Cadence per Minute)**	**Land Running (Min/Mile)**
1	Very light (< 50)	Slow walk (> 21)
2	Light (50 to 60)	Medium-paced walk (15 to 20)
3	Somewhat hard (60 to 75)	Fast walk/jog (< 15)
4	Hard (75 to 85)	Run (5 to 10)
5	Very hard (> 85)	Very hard run (< 5)

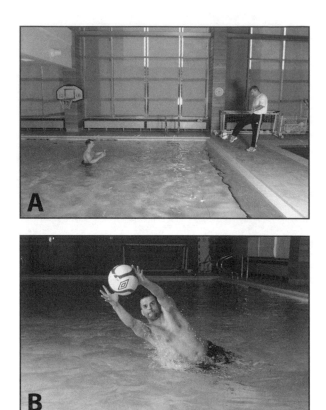

Figure 4-55. (A) Sport and (B) position-specific drills can be incorporated into the athlete's aquatic program prior to initiation into land-based drills. (Reprinted with permission from Jason Palmer, BHMS (Ed) Hons, BPhty, MCSP.)

rate.[28] Cadence can be controlled using an auditory metronome. Heart rate responses can then be recorded at varying levels of cadence, which can provide the expected heart rate and physiologic response for a given cadence level. This can allow for a designed workout based on time intervals for a given cadence level. Table 4-1 can be used to convert cadence rates to a running pace on land. To allow the practitioner to monitor progression, the speed of movement can be assessed by stride frequency. This can be assessed in 30- to 60-sec intervals as the patient sprints and the number of strides achieved is monitored. When monitoring exercise intensity, the heart rate is used primarily during extended runs, and the rating of perceived exertion and cadence rates are more often used for sprint and interval training.[26]

RETURN TO SPORT

The final stage of the rehabilitation process is that of returning to training or playing. The goal of the rehab process is to ensure that an athlete is ready to be reintroduced to the training environment in a safe manner and is not at unnecessary risk of breakdown because the rehab process has not "ticked all the boxes" along the way. Like progression of function during the rehab process, reintroduction to the training or playing environment should be seen as the natural next step of progression. If this step seems a little too big, either the nature of the reintroduction needs to be considered—that is, modified training—or more steps need to be included. In team sports, for example, particularly after a lengthy time out due to significant injury, often it is better if the rehab process has pushed the athlete beyond the physical demands of what will be required in the training environment. Thus, when the athlete is reintroduced back to team-based work, he or she can focus on the stimulus of sessions with multiple players around him or her and

the associated demands rather than having to do this and being physically challenged at the same time, which may be too great a step to take at once. Therefore, it is important to attempt to simulate all specific sporting activities and demands in order to prepare an athlete to return to his sporting activity (Figure 4-55). This preparation needs to consider not only the various movement patterns inherent to the activity to be undertaken but also the conditioning status of the athlete. Proper conditioning during aquatic therapy can be made easier if the trainer uses a pool with an underwater treadmill and embedded video monitor to evaluate and correct gait patterns before they become problematic or symptomatic. This will also allow a patient to gain confidence in the activities and movements while also allowing some possibly needed extra healing time. Through adjustment of pool depths, activity speeds, and the progression from basic to high-level function, the water can be used effectively to bridge the gap between nonweight-bearing function to full weight-bearing function.

When applicable, the patient should also begin gradually implementing land impact activities that are ready to be progressed from the water. As mentioned above, once a patient can perform an activity with quality at 50% weight bearing, he or she is ready for this activity to be introduced full weight bearing in its most basic form. These progressions can occur throughout the rehab process, such that water- and land-based work can be included in a single day's or week's program until the patient is ready for full function on land. However, before returning to a full land functional activity program, the patient should be able to perform all sports-specific training and testing in the water without any signs of pain, swelling, or soreness. This also ensures that the athlete is not returned too quickly to his or her prior level without allowing ample time for healing.

Once returning to land-based functional activity/ training, the athlete may still choose to continue to incorporate aquatic therapy into his or her training program on a periodic basis to assist in the prevention of overuse injuries and impact loading and provide a mental training break. As a University of Wisconsin–Eau Claire Department of Kinesiology study[29] concluded, when 2×/week hydrotherapy sessions on an underwater treadmill were added to land-based exercise of healthy, active adults, no subjects experienced adverse effects from the additional days of exercise. However, many did receive physical and psychological benefits, including 20% improvement in hamstring flexibility after approximately 5 weeks; a postexercise fatigue drop from 1.8/10 to 0.6/10 over 5 weeks; better quality of sleep; and a drop in muscle/joint pain/soreness 2 to 4 hours postexercise during the course of the program.

CLINICAL OUTCOMES

The outcome of any rehabilitation program is judged by how effectively and efficiently treatment goals are achieved throughout and at the end of the rehab process. Aquatic therapy, including that which is performed on an underwater treadmill, has been shown to be an effective form of exercise in the treatment of various lower extremity conditions. Tovin et al reported that following an 8-week program following ACL reconstruction surgery, patients undergoing an aquatic-based program compared to a land-based program had less joint effusion, reported greater functional improvement, and had higher Lysholm scores.[9] Another study, authored by Sanders and Lawson,[30] found that patients who had intraarticular ACL reconstructions and who participated in 12 weeks of water-based aquatic therapy in a pool with an underwater treadmill (versus those who participated in 12 weeks of land-based therapy alone) showed a greater minimization of joint effusion and self-reported greater functional improvements. These findings led the study authors to conclude that all phases of ACL rehabilitation could be safely undertaken in an aquatic environment.

Aquatic therapy has been shown to be superior to land-based exercise in relieving pain before and after a 50-ft walk test.[31] When comparing a land-based exercise program to an aquatic exercise program, Wyatt and coworkers reported no significant difference in knee ROM, thigh girth, and 1-mile walk time; however the subjective pain levels were significantly less in the aquatic group.[32] Himan et al reported that subjects having either hip or knee osteoarthritis who underwent a 6-week aquatic program reported less pain and joint stiffness, greater physical function, quality of life, and hip muscle strength compared to a group of controls.[33] In a Utah State University[34] research study that evaluated underwater treadmill exercise in patients with osteoarthritis of the knee, hip, or ankle, patients reported that their perceived pain was 140% greater during land treadmill exercise sessions than during underwater treadmill exercise sessions. These findings support anecdotal reports from athletes in a variety of sports who have undergone aquatic therapy using underwater treadmills.

CONCLUSION

Water is an environment that offers many benefits in injury treatment and rehabilitation for lower extremity pathology. Compared to land-based rehabilitation, water's qualities of increased hydrostatic pressure, increased viscosity, and buoyancy, to name just a few, can make water a superior therapy environment at various stages of the rehab progress. When combined with the latest technology of underwater treadmills, water jets, and video monitoring, it is clear that aquatic therapy can significantly enhance therapy for any patient at any stage of his rehabilitation.

REFERENCES

1. Harrison RN, Lees A, McCullagh PJ, Rowe WB. A bioengineering analysis of human muscle and joint forces in the lower limbs during running. *J Sports Sci* 1986;4(3):201-218.
2. Flynn TW, Soutas-Little RW. Patellofemoral joint compressive forces in forward and backward running. *J Orthop Sports Phys Ther.* 1995;21(5):277-282.
3. Morrison JB. The mechanics of the knee joint in relation to normal walking. *J Biomech.* 1970;3(1):51-61.
4. Pantoja PD, Alberton CL, Pilla C, Vendrusculo AP, Kruel LF. Effect of resistive exercise on muscle damage in water and on land. *J Strength Cond Res.* 2009;23:1051-1054.
5. Levin S. Aquatic therapy. *Phys Sportsmed.* 1991;19(10):119-126.
6. Speer K, Cavanaugh JT, Warren RF, Day L, Wickiewicz TL. A role for hydrotherapy in shoulder rehabilitation. *Am J Sports Med.* 1993;21:850-853.
7. Herring SA. Rehabilitation of muscle injuries. *Med Sci Sports Exerc.* 1990;22:453-456.
8. Rivera JE. Open versus closed kinetic chain rehabilitation of the lower extremity: a functional and biomechanical analysis. *J Sport Rehabil.* 1994;3:154-167.
9. Tovin BJ, Wolf SL, Greenfield BH, Crouse J, Woodfin BA. Comparison of the effects of exercise in water and on land on the rehabilitation of patients with intra articular anterior cruciate ligament reconstruction. *Phys Ther.* 1994;74:710-719.
10. Noyes FR. Functional properties of knee ligaments and alteration induced by immobilization. *Clin Orthop.* 1977;123:210-242.
11. Cole AJ, Eagleston RE, Moschetti M, et al. Spine pain: aquatic rehabilitation strategies. *J Back Musculoskel Rehabil.* 1994;4:273.

12. Salazar A, Dolny D. Underwater Treadmill Running: The Low Impact, Pain Free, Calorie Burning Fitness Advantage. Middletown, PA: HydroWorx; 2012.

13. Malone TR, Garret WE, Zachazewki JE. Muscle: Deformation, injury, repair. In: Zachazewski JE, Magee DJ, Quillen WS, eds. *Athletic Injuries and Rehabilitation*. Philadelphia, PA: W.B. Saunders Company; 1996:71-91.

14. Pöyhönen T, Keskinen KL, Hautala A, Savolainen J, Mälkiä A. Human isometric force production and electromyogram activity of knee extensors muscles in water and on dry land. *Eur J Appl Physiol Occup Physiol*. 1999;80:52-56.

15. Pöyhönen T, Kyröläinen H, Keskinen KL, Hautala A, Savolainen J, Mälkiä A. Electromyographic and kinematic analysis of therapeutic knee exercises under water. *Clin Biomech*. 2001;16:496-504.

16. Frey LA, Smidt GL. Underwater forces produced by the Hydro-Tone Bell. *J Orthop Sports Phys Ther*. 1996;23:267-271.

17. Visnic MA. Aquatic physical therapy comes of age. *Aquatic Phys Ther Reports*. 1994;1:6-8.

18. Pöyhönen T, Keskinen KL, Kyröläinen H, Hautala A, Savolainen J, Mälkiä A. Neuromuscular function during therapeutic knee exercise under water and on dry land. *Arch Phys Med Rehabil*. 2001;82:1446-1452.

19. Triplett NT, Colado JC, Benavent J, et al. Concentric and impact forces of single-leg jumps in an aquatic environment versus on land. *Med Sci Sports Exerc*. 2009;41:1790-1796.

20. Martel GF, Harmer ML, Logan JM, Parker CB. Aquatic plyometric training increases vertical jump in female volleyball players. *Med Sci Sports Exerc*. 2005;37:1814-1819.

21. Khalid W, Amin M, Boben T. The influence of the upper extremity movement on take-off in vertical jump. In: Tsarouchas L, Teraudi B, Gowistzke B, Holt L, eds. *Biomechanics in Sports V*. Athens, Greece: Hellenic Sports Research Institute; 1989:375-379

22. Lees A, Barton G. The interpretation of relative momentum data to access the contribution of the force limbs to the generation of vertical velocity in sports activities. *J Sports Sci*. 1996;14:503-511.

23. Harrison AJ, Moroney A. Arm augmentation of vertical jump performance in young girls and adult females. Paper presented at: XXV ISBS Symposium; 2007, Ouro Preto, Brazil.

24. Feltner ME, Fraschetti DJ, Crisp RJ. Upper extremity augmentation of lower extremity kinetics during countermovement vertical jumps. *J Sports Sci*. 1999;17:449-466.

25. Feltner ME, Bishop EJ, Perez CM. Segmental and kinetic contributions in vertical jumps performed with and without an arm swing. *Res Q Exerc Sport*. 2004;75:216-230.

26. Wilder RP, Brennan D. Aqua running for athletic rehabilitation. In: O'Conner F, Wilder R, eds. *The Textbook of Running Medicine*. New York, NY: McGraw Hill; 2001.

27. Brennan DK, Wilder RP. *Aqua Running: An Instructor's Manual*. Houston, TX: Houston International Running Center; 1990.

28. Wilder RP, Brennan D, Schotte DE. A standard measure for exercise prescription for aqua running. *Am J Sports Med*. 1993;21:45-48.

29. Desmond A, Bayliss A, Jacobsen H, Hardy H, Jarvey K, Bredle D. *Health Benefits of Underwater Treadmill Exercise for Active Adults*. Eau Claire, WI: University of Wisconsin; 2010.

30. Sanders M, Lawson B. In the pool: knee anterior cruciate ligament recovery program. *ACSMs Health Fit J*. 2010;14:34-35.

31. Silva LE, Valim V, Pessanha AP, et al. Hydrotherapy versus conventional land-based exercise for the management of patients with osteoarthritis of the knee: a randomized clinical trial. *Phys Ther*. 2008;88:12-21.

32. Wyatt FB, Milam S, Manske RC, Deere R. The effects of aquatic and traditional exercise programs on persons with knee osteoarthritis. *J Strength Cond Res*. 2001;15:337-340.

33. Hinman RS, Heywood SE, Day AR. Aquatic therapy for hip and knee osteoarthritis: results of a single-blind randomized controlled trial. *Phys Ther*. 2007;87:32-43.

34. Denning WM, Bressel E, Dolny D. Underwater treadmill exercise as a potential treatment for adults with osteoarthritis. *IJARE*. 2010;4:70-80.

Aquatic Application for the Upper Extremity

Leonard C. Macrina, MSPT, SCS, CSCS; A. J. Yenchak, PT, DPT, CSCS;
Kevin E. Wilk, PT, DPT, FAPTA; and Mike Reinold, DPT, ATC, CSCS

The shoulder, elbow, wrist, and hand are complex structures vulnerable to a variety of injuries occurring either from a traumatic event or through repetitive, overuse activities. Postinjury rehabilitation can be a daunting task and an intimidating time for a patient. The thought of inactivity related to injury and or uncertainty in postsurgical plans of care can create emotional, psychological, and physical barriers that may hinder rehabilitative progression and outcome. Aquatic therapy for the shoulder, elbow, wrist, and hand serves as an integral technique in the field of sports medicine, work-related injury, and general rehabilitation. Although aquatic rehabilitation appears to make its greatest contribution in the treatment of impairments to the hip, knee, and shoulder, the benefits of elbow, wrist, and hand aquatic rehabilitation may be underestimated. Combinations of multiplanar functional movement patterns of the shoulder, elbow, wrist, and hand can be assimilated during aquatic rehabilitation to improve range of motion (ROM), progress strength, aid in regaining neuromuscular control/proprioception, and promote muscular endurance.

Aquatic therapy can be used in conjunction with land-based therapy programs to further enhance restoration of motion, reduce muscle spasm, and aid in integrating dynamic movement patterns to enhance tissue healing and functional recovery. Early in the rehabilitation process, the rehabilitation specialist may consider both land- and water-based therapy to quickly and safely return the patient to his prior level of function.[1,2] Aquatic therapy may provide a supportive medium during which protective active movements may begin at an earlier stage in the rehabilitation process compared to land-based therapy.[3]

Aquatic therapy is a safe and beneficial form of exercise. In addition to a number of cardiovascular and respiratory benefits, Table 5-1 shows other potential benefits of aquatic therapy. The use of aquatic therapy as it relates to hydrostatic pressure, viscosity, and water depth may be a useful adjunct modality in the successful rehabilitation of upper extremity injuries.[1-8]

The healing benefits of water immersion and principles of hydrostatic pressure have been exemplified for centuries. Thermal mineral water immersion has resulted in peripheral edema reduction, enhanced joint mobility, and decreased joint pain, which can aid in restoration of motion of the shoulder, elbow, wrist, and hand. Temperature changes related to warm or cold water create vascular responses that either dilate or constrict blood vessels. Warm water may be beneficial for preparing upper extremity musculature for stretching exercises by decreasing gamma motor excitation and increasing blood flow to aid in healing and improve extensibility.[8,9] Cold water may slow cellular metabolic rates related to inflammation.[10]

Water depth is a crucial aspect of aquatic therapy when prescribing rehabilitation programs for patients. As water depth increases, hydrostatic pressure and buoyancy increase, resulting in compromised stability of the patient. This may be detrimental when prescribing an exercise protocol for a postoperative patient or someone with a balance disorder. Water levels should be carefully monitored, especially in the early stages of aquatic rehabilitation when performing upright exercises related to the shoulder, elbow, wrist, and hand. Proper execution of movements is dependent on posturing of the individual at a desired depth of water immersion. For successful management and

Wilk KE, Joyner DM. *The Use of Aquatics in Orthopedic and Sports Medicine Rehabilitation and Physical Conditioning (pp 61-70).*
© 2014 SLACK Incorporated.

Table 5-1.

Potential Benefits of Aquatic Therapy

- Increase and maintain muscular flexibility
- Improve mobility and ROM
- Increase muscular strength
- Improve coordination, balance, and postural alignment

rehabilitation of shoulder, elbow, wrist, and hand pathology, appropriate water depths should be utilized based on posture and alignment, the individual's skill level, and safety precautions. Optimal exercise depths will fully submerge the affected joint(s).

The purpose of this chapter is to review the principles of aquatic-based shoulder, elbow, wrist, and hand rehabilitation; assess epidemiology related to elbow, wrist, and hand pathology; provide a framework of rehabilitative concepts to aid the health care provider in nonoperative/operative procedure; and outline specific aquatic exercises that may be beneficial in the promotion/restoration of shoulder, elbow, wrist, and hand function.

AQUATIC REHABILITATION FOR THE SHOULDER

Shoulder pathology, particularly to the rotator cuff, is common in the orthopedic outpatient population. Nonoperative and postoperative rehabilitation is often utilized to restore the patient's function. The rehabilitation process must include the restoration of ROM, muscular strength, muscular endurance, as well as a gradual restoration of proprioception, dynamic stability, and neuromuscular control.

Careful progression of ROM and strength is initiated early on in the rehabilitation process. A key tool to early rehabilitation is the use of aquatic therapy. More commonly, aquatic therapy is utilized as part of the rehabilitation process after surgery to the hip and knee joints. There are few studies documenting the electromyographic (EMG) activity of the shoulder musculature in the pool,[11-13] although existing studies demonstrated a substantial decrease in muscle activation compared to dry land exercise. Functional stability of the glenohumeral joint is accomplished through the integrated functions of the joint capsule, ligaments, and glenoid labrum, as well as the neuromuscular control and dynamic stabilization of the surrounding musculature, particularly the rotator cuff muscles.[14-18] Dynamic stabilization of the glenohumeral joint is achieved through the interaction of several active mechanisms. The muscles primarily involved include the rotator cuff, deltoid, and biceps brachii.[19,20] Secondary stabilizers include the pectoralis major, latissimus dorsi, and scapulothoracic musculature (trapezius group, rhomboids, serratus anterior, pectoralis minor, levator scapulae). Exercises to promote early activation in a safe manner may be accomplished in the water.

The rotator cuff has been shown to be a substantial dynamic stabilizer of the glenohumeral joint in multiple shoulder positions.[21] Appropriate rehabilitation progression and strengthening of the rotator cuff muscles are important in order to provide appropriate force to help elevate and move the arm, compress and center the humeral head within the glenoid fossa during shoulder movements, and resist humeral head superior translation due to deltoid activity.[22-27] The surrounding stabilizing structures play a vital role in dynamically stabilizing the overhead athlete's shoulder joint due to the excessive mobility inherent to this population.[18,28,29] This allows the glenohumeral joint musculature to produce and dissipate the large forces that are generated during overhead movements. Deficiency of these muscle groups may lead to a variety of injuries to the labrum capsule or rotator cuff.

The unique properties of water, including buoyancy, viscosity, and hydrostatic pressure, allow for patients to perform activities with less stress. Viscosity is defined as the resistance of the water by means of gentle friction, allowing strengthening and conditioning of an injury while reducing the risk of further injury. The unique principles of buoyancy within the water are utilized as therapeutic exercises are prescribed for various shoulder pathologies. The effects of hydrostatic pressure on the patient include improved heart and lung function, making aquatic exercise a useful way to maintain and strengthen cardiovascular function along with the many benefits during upper extremity rehabilitation. This pressure effect also aids in improving muscle blood flow that may aid in tissue healing and extensibility.[30] In this chapter we have included numerous rehabilitation protocols in the appendices to help facilitate aquatic exercise for the upper extremity. Appendix F, G, and H illustrate these exercises. ROM exercises may be better performed in the pool, especially if the patient exhibits apprehension or muscle guarding. Examples include a patient with an acutely dislocated shoulder joint or a patient with spasms as a result of adhesive capsulitis. The water's buoyancy aids in upward movement of the glenohumeral joint, which can assist in improving the patient's overall function. By definition, buoyancy is the upward force caused by fluid pressure that keeps things afloat. The net upward buoyancy force is equal to the magnitude of the weight of fluid displaced by the body. This force enables the object to float or at least seem lighter. Although the water's buoyancy is critical to allowing for early exercise, other concepts should also be considered when putting together an appropriate exercise program. Other variables include (1) direction of movement within the water, (2) lever arm length, (3) water depth, and (4) weighted or flotation equipment used[31] (Table 5-2).

Table 5-2.

Variables to Consider When Utilizing Aquatic Therapy

- Buoyancy

- Direction of movement

- Length of lever arm

- Water depth

- Weight or flotation device being used

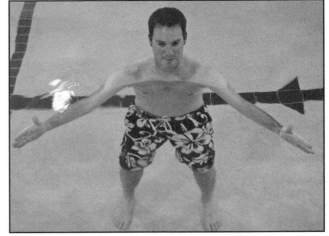

Figure 5-1. Assisted shoulder flexion in a standing position using the water's buoyancy. (Reprinted with permission from Leonard C. Macrina, MSPT, SCS, CSCS.)

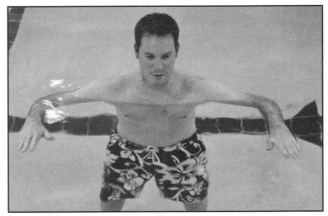

Figure 5-3. Shorter lever arm abduction is more stressful on the shoulder joint's soft tissue structures. (Reprinted with permission from Leonard C. Macrina, MSPT, SCS, CSCS.)

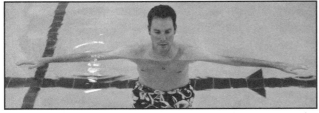

Figure 5-2. Assisted shoulder abduction in a standing position utilizing the water's buoyancy properties. (Reprinted with permission from Leonard C. Macrina, MSPT, SCS, CSCS.)

Active ROM (AROM) activities are permitted when adequate muscular strength and balance have been achieved. When prescribing activities within the water, the clinician should be aware that the exercise can be buoyancy assisted or resisted. Initially, the patient can begin with submaximal, pain-free isometrics for shoulder flexion, extension, abduction, external rotation, internal rotation, and elbow flexion. Isometrics are used to hinder muscular atrophy and restore voluntary muscular control while avoiding detrimental shoulder forces. Isometrics should be performed at multiple angles throughout the available ROM. Particular emphasis is placed on contraction at the end of the currently available ROM. In addition, a patient with painful adhesive capsulitis may be able to perform AROM activities with less pain, guarding, and muscle spasms.

A movement toward the surface of the water, such as shoulder flexion (elevation; Figure 5-1) or abduction, is considered buoyancy assisted. Altering the lever arm length can affect the amount of resistance or assistance that the water is providing to the extremity. For example, shoulder abduction with the elbow extended (Figure 5-2) is considered more buoyancy assisted than with the elbow flexed (Figure 5-3). For a postoperative patient in whom the forces need to be minimized, the patient should initiate buoyancy-assisted activities with longer lever arms and progress to short lever arm motions. ROM exercises are performed immediately in a restricted ROM based on the theory that motion assists in the enhancement and organization of collagen tissue and the stimulation of joint mechanoreceptors and may assist in the neuromodulation of pain. The

rehabilitation program should allow for progressive applied loads, beginning with gentle passive ROM. A movement that is parallel to the bottom of the pool, such as horizontal shoulder abduction (Figure 5-4) or horizontal adduction, is not considered resistive or assisted by the water's buoyancy. This type of movement may be utilized shortly after initiating buoyancy-assisted activities and before beginning resistance-type movements.

On the other hand, activities such as shoulder extension (Figure 5-5) and adduction are considered buoyancy resisted due to the downwardly directed movements. These activities should be incorporated once adequate tissue healing has occurred and can be performed without any pain or discomfort.

The water's depth will greatly affect the forces on the shoulder joint. Varying the patient's standing depth will control the amount of movement available on the joint. Early on in the rehabilitation process, flotation equipment may be used to aid in assisted movements and decrease stresses on the shoulder joint (Figure 5-6). As the patient gains ROM and tissue healing proceeds, positioning may be altered to include above shoulder-height ROM exercises.

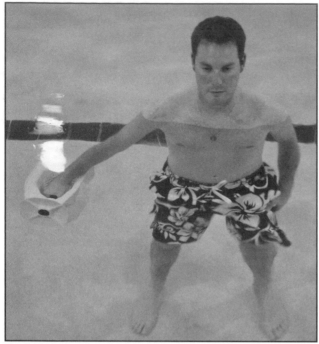

Figure 5-4. Standing shoulder horizontal abduction using the resistance of the water to aid in muscle activation. (Reprinted with permission from Leonard C. Macrina, MSPT, SCS, CSCS.)

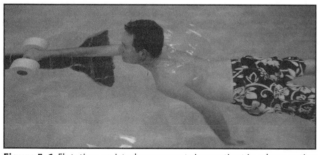

Figure 5-6. Flotation-assisted movements in a patient in whom active movements may be contraindicated. (Reprinted with permission from Leonard C. Macrina, MSPT, SCS, CSCS.)

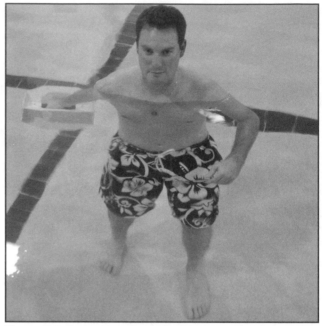

Figure 5-5. Buoyancy-resisted shoulder extension in standing. (Reprinted with permission from Leonard C. Macrina, MSPT, SCS, CSCS.)

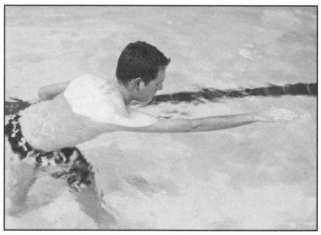

Figure 5-7. Bent forward at the waist for overhead flexion assisted by the water's buoyancy. (Reprinted with permission from Leonard C. Macrina, MSPT, SCS, CSCS.)

The patient may perform movements in supine for abduction or standing bent forward at the waist for overhead flexion (Figure 5-7). The patient may also float on his or her back while holding the edge of the pool, the rail, or a flotation device to work on the overhead position. Once the patient advances, this position may also be utilized as a stretching technique for the upper extremity. The warm water and buoyancy may make stretching easier to perform due to improved tissue extensibility and relaxation of surrounding musculature.

If tolerated by the patient, exercises in a prone position while wearing a flotation device may also be incorporated to promote overhead flexion (Figure 5-8). In this position, gentle strengthening through the water's resistance may be incorporated through long lever arm motions or with handheld paddles. In a standing position, the patient may perform external and internal rotation at 0 degrees of abduction, similar to a land-based exercise utilizing exercise tubing (Figure 5-9). EMG studies have shown that this exercise strengthens the infraspinatus and teres minor.[20]

In addition, the full can exercise (Figure 5-10) may be the most beneficial exercise and provides the least amount of pain provocation from an anatomical and biomechanical standpoint due to the increased amount of subacromial space[32-34] and increased moment arm of the supraspinatus muscle[21,35,36] in the standing position. This exercise has been shown to best isolate the supraspinatus muscle with minimal surrounding muscle activation.[12,19,20,22] Kelly et al[12] further showed that lower normalized integrated EMG amplitude about the shoulder when slow (30 degrees/sec and 45 degrees/sec) shoulder elevation was performed in the scapular plane in water compared to the same movement performed on dry land.

Patients who perform upper extremity exercises in the pool find many other benefits. Trunk muscle cocontraction occurs, which benefits the core while also working

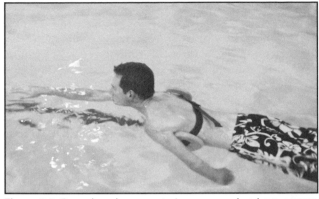

Figure 5-8. Prone long lever arm to improve overhead movements. (Reprinted with permission from Leonard C. Macrina, MSPT, SCS, CSCS.)

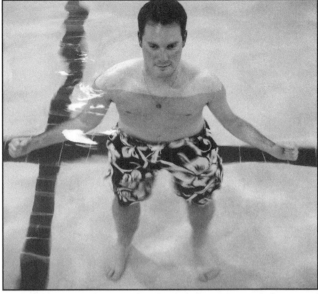

Figure 5-9. Resisted external and internal rotation at 0 degrees of abduction to enhance rotator cuff strengthening. (Reprinted with permission from Leonard C. Macrina, MSPT, SCS, CSCS.)

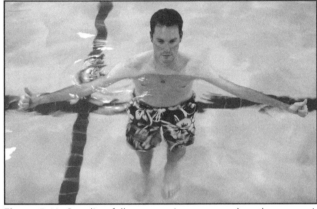

Figure 5-10. Standing full can exercise to strengthen the supraspinatus muscle. (Reprinted with permission from Leonard C. Macrina, MSPT, SCS, CSCS.)

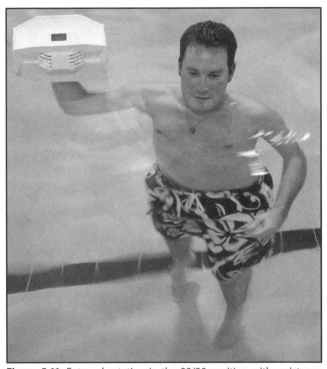

Figure 5-11. External rotation in the 90/90 position with resistance from the water to promote functional rotator cuff strengthening in the throwing position. (Reprinted with permission from Leonard C. Macrina, MSPT, SCS, CSCS.)

on balance and stability. AROM activities, including proprioceptive neuromuscular facilitation (PNF) patterns and 90/90 resistance (Figure 5-11), serve to simultaneously activate hip and abdominal musculature while strengthening the shoulder in a functional position. Lower extremity, core, and trunk strength are critical to efficiently perform overhead activities by transferring and dissipating forces in a coordinated fashion. Core stabilization drills are utilized to further enhance proximal stability with distal mobility of the upper extremity. Core stabilization is used based on the kinetic chain concept where imbalance within any point of the kinetic chain may result in pathology throughout. To efficiently perform movement patterns such as throwing requires a precise interaction of the entire body kinetic chain. An imbalance of strength, flexibility, endurance, and stability may result in fatigue, abnormal arthrokinematics, and subsequent compensation.

The patient can also perform closed kinetic chain activities, which will enhance rotator cuff activation through cocontraction[37-39] and improve proprioception[28,37,39-41] as the patient stabilizes. The goal of this is to stimulate articular receptors and facilitate cocontraction of the shoulder force couples, thus incorporating a combination of eccentric and concentric contractions to provide joint stability. While in a supine position the patient may perform overhead push-pull motions utilizing the resistance from the water and progress to holding aquatic equipment for added resistance. Dips or push-ups can also be performed at the pool's edge by varying the depth of the water in which the patient is standing. An excellent stability exercise involves the patient floating in the prone position and pressing flotation equipment toward the bottom of the pool.[8] Initially the patient may utilize both hands and then progress to the involved extremity as strength and neuromuscular control improve.

Sports-specific movements may also be simulated in the pool as an adjunct to land-based movements. A baseball player may swing an old baseball bat or a tennis player may use an old racket to reproduce the swinging motion. Various pieces of aquatic equipment may be utilized to simulate the sports-specific movement but also create significant resistance while performing the act in the water.

Epidemiology and Aquatic Rehabilitation for the Elbow, Wrist, and Hand

Epidemiology of Elbow, Wrist, and Hand Injuries

The elbow, wrist, and hand are susceptible to injury due to their crucial role in daily function, work-related activity, and athletics. The type of injury depends on intrinsic and extrinsic variables (age, tissue quality, ligamentous laxity), environment in which the patient performs the activity, and the task to be performed.

Acute injuries to the elbow such as fracture, dislocation, and sprain/strain result from falls onto an outstretched arm. Frostick and Safran have reported that radial head fractures account for approximately one third of all elbow fractures.[42,43]

Safran suggested that elbow injuries are becoming more prevalent in people who participate in throwing and racquet sports.[43]

Injuries can be categorized into enthesopathies such as medial/lateral epicondylitis, valgus stress injury, chondral abnormalities related to overhead athletes, and nerve compression syndromes.[42,43]

Osteochondritis dissecans, osteophytic spurring of the olecranon process, radiocapitellar compression syndrome, and elbow apophysitis are closely related to pathology found in the thrower's elbow. Tullos and King[44] reported that 50% of baseball pitchers have injuries to either the shoulder or elbow that prevent them from performing at some point in their career.[42-44]

In baseball pitchers, most elbow injuries occur in the late cocking and early acceleration phase of throwing. Excessive tensile force is placed on the ulnar collateral ligament (UCL) of the medial elbow, and compressive forces are transmitted through the radiocapitellar joint and olecranon, termed *valgus extension overload*.[42,43,45,46] These forces can ultimately lead to failure of the UCL, osteochondral fracture of the radiocapitellar joint, and osteophytic change on the posterior olecranon. Chondral compression/valgus stress injuries can also occur in other sports, such as gymnastics, tennis, and golf.

Gymnasts can transmit high forces throughout their upper body during tumbling, balance, and handstand posturing, which can ultimately lead to breakdown of medial elbow ligaments and soft tissue. Tumbling exercises require high triceps force output. Repetitive flexion, extension, and loading of the elbow can lead to inflammation of the triceps insertion, osteochondral defects, and ulnar nerve traction injury. Jackson et al reported 10 cases of osteochondritis dissecans of the capitellum in 7 elite gymnasts, with only one gymnast training at a 2.9-year follow-up.[47]

Tennis players can develop chronic conditions of their forearm flexor/extensor mechanism secondary to overuse (lateral epicondylitis). Morris et al found that the pronator teres and triceps musculature aid in power production during serving.[48] Kibler demonstrated that the elbow joint contributes to 15% of the total force output during the tennis serve.[49] He concluded that the motion for ground strokes creates smaller torques on the elbow. However, the term *tennis elbow* can be misleading, in that 95% of cases of lateral epicondylitis occur in non-tennis players, including golfers, athletes, workers, and musicians.[50] Lateral epicondylitis involves degeneration of the origin of the extensor carpi radialis brevis (ECRB) tendon at its insertion on the lateral epicondyle. Pathology related to this diagnosis may not be inflammatory in nature. Histological studies have shown that cellular markers for inflammation are not present in the origin of the tendon with those that are symptomatic at or near the insertion of the ECRB. Tendon pathology may be the result of gradual degradation with tendon thinning, increased cellularity, nonuniformity of collagen fibers, and an abundance of fibroblasts. Therefore, tendonitis, tendonosis, chronic tendon injury, and tendonopathy cannot be used synonymously.

Medial epicondylitis (golfers elbow) refers to tendon pathology related to the flexor/pronator muscle origin. It is far less common than its counterpart, tennis elbow, and involves repetitive valgus strain on the medial elbow. Over 80% of cases involve men and commonly occur in the right arm of a right-handed golfer.[43]

Wrist and hand injuries are common in sport and the workplace. Rettig[50] proposed that overuse tendon injuries can create colossal costs in the workplace and they account for approximately 30% to 50% of all sports injuries. The types of injuries range from traumatic fractures seen in contact sports such as hockey to overuse, repetitive injuries in gymnastics, golf, racquet sports, musicians, artists, and desk occupations. Wrist and hand injuries are more common in adolescents than adults. Over a 10-year period, the Cleveland Clinic found that 14.8% of athletic patients under the age of 16 sustained upper extremity injuries, and 9% involved the wrist.[50]

Work-related musculoskeletal disorders of the hand and wrist are associated with the longest absences from work and are therefore associated with the greatest loss of productivity and wages compared to injuries to any other anatomical region according to Barr and colleagues.[51] Pathophysiology parallels that of overuse tendonopathy and chronic nerve compression injury. Risk factors for overuse syndromes include repetition, high force, joint posture, direct pressure, and vibration. Common overuse syndromes include trigger finger, carpal tunnel syndrome, de Quervain syndrome, and gamekeepers thumb.

Trigger finger can be defined as a narrowing stenosis or fibrosis of the tendon sheath in the affected finger. This condition is normally caused by repetitive gripping activities. Nodules form on the tendon sheath secondary to chronic inflammation and impede anatomical gliding of the respective tendon. Carpal tunnel syndrome entails compression of the median nerve as it traverses the wrist. Symptoms include numbness and tingling in the median nerve distribution of the hand, which involves both volar/dorsal side symptoms. De Quervain syndrome is an idiopathic degenerative disorder of the tendons extensor pollicis brevis and abductor pollicis longus. Symptoms normally involve pain along the radial side of the wrist with repetitive thumb motions. Some have likened this injury to repetitive use of Blackberry cell phones, also known as Blackberry thumb.[52] Gamekeepers thumb involves injury to the UCL of the thumb, resulting in instability. This injury can manifest as an acute injury in skiers falling on an outstretched hand or a chronic condition of repetitive hyperabduction of the thumb.

The Bureau of Labor Statistics (BLS) keeps record of occupational illnesses and injury that occur in private industry.[53] In 1999 the BLS reported 73,195 repetitive motion injuries, 44,504 of which were related to tendonosis and carpal tunnel syndrome. Incidence rates for tendonosis and carpal tunnel syndrome were 1 in every 2000 private industry workers. Average days missed from work were also calculated. Tendonosis accounted for an average of 17 days of absenteeism and carpal tunnel syndrome demonstrated a much higher absenteeism rate of 27 in 1999. The BLS has also reported that women account for 33% of the total number of injuries in private industry jobs in 1999. Women incurred 65% of the total tendonosis and carpal tunnel syndrome injuries in 1999. The incidence of these injuries are higher in women than men partly because more women have jobs requiring repetitive motion, because equipment is ergonomically manufactured to male body types, and due to possible tissue histological structuring (higher type III collagen).

Understanding pathology related to the elbow, wrist, and hand aids the rehabilitation specialist in promoting safe, effective, and therapeutic exercise prescriptions for patients who sustain these injuries. Being able to accurately diagnose and treat these injuries should be a collaborative effort headed by physicians, physical therapists, and athletic trainers. Communication among these professionals will outline a plan of care that is unique and individualized to the patient's needs, incorporate work/athletic/general movement patterns that are functional and safe to perform, and follow a progressive multiphase approach to rehabilitating the injury. Aquatic therapy provides an excellent medium for the restoration of motion and function to the elbow, wrist, and hand. Principles of water immersion have been applied to help in the healing and reestablishment of homeostasis of injured tissue.

Aquatic Rehabilitation Approach

Aquatic rehabilitation following elbow, wrist, and hand injury or surgery follows an ordered and progressive multiphase approach. The goal of any nonoperative or postsurgical aquatic rehabilitation regimen is to return the patient to his or her prior level of function safely and in a timely manner. Rehabilitation of the elbow, wrist, and hand stresses the restoration of motion, regaining strength, and developing neuromuscular control. The 4 phases of operative/nonoperative aquatic rehabilitation are to (1) protect healing structures while restoring motion, (2) enhance mobility of the affected joints, (3) develop strength and proprioception, and (4) return the patient to sport/occupation. The rehabilitation specialist must assess the patient's condition to ensure that treatment is effective, reliable, accurate, and appropriate for the patient's stage of healing. ROM exercises are used to help regain mobility, decrease pain, and control swelling. Phase 2 emphasizes facilitation of strength/proprioceptive exercises, advanced mobility, stabilization, and endurance activities. Phase 3 incorporates advanced strengthening exercises that incorporate ROM, strength, and stability. Phase 4 is the last step of this 4-phase model that prepares the patient for return to sport/occupation, which consists of sport-specific or work-simulated tasks. Listed below are the 4 phases of aquatic rehabilitation utilized to treat pathology related to the elbow, wrist, and hand.

Phase 1—Restoring Range of Motion

The first phase in aquatic rehabilitation of the elbow, wrist, and hand is restoring ROM. This phase emphasizes minimizing the effects of immobilization, decreasing pain and inflammation, regaining ROM, and minimizing muscle atrophy. ROM exercises are performed to nourish articular cartilage and aid in the genesis, alignment, and organization of collagen. Exercises are performed for all elbow and wrist motions to prevent the negative effects of scar tissue/adhesion formation. AROM and passive ROM exercises are performed on the humeroulnar, humeroradial, and radioulnar joints to restore flexion/extension (Figure 5-12) and supination/pronation, respectively. Hand dexterity is also emphasized, with an emphasis on gripping. Early AROM and passive ROM of the humeroulnar joint aids in reducing the occurrence of elbow flexion contractures. According to Wilk et al, the elbow joint has the ability to develop flexion contractures based on the congruency of the joint, lack of capsular redundancy, and the sensitivity of the anterior capsule to stress.[46,54] The brachialis muscle also crosses the anterior aspect of the elbow joint with capsular connections. Injury to the elbow may cause adhesion/scar tissue formation of the brachialis, further limiting motion.[54]

Secondary goals of this phase of rehabilitation include ridding the joint of pain and inflammation. Cold water

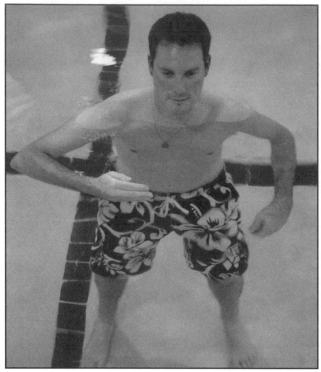

Figure 5-12. Active-assisted elbow flexion and extension. (Reprinted with permission from Leonard C. Macrina, MSPT, SCS, CSCS.)

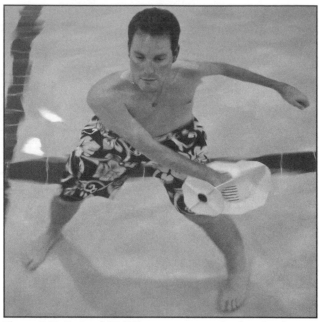

Figure 5-13. Resisted D2 PNF patterns promoting functional movement patterns. (Reprinted with permission from Leonard C. Macrina, MSPT, SCS, CSCS.)

immersion can aid in the slowing of metabolic processes related to inflammation, and warm water can aid blood flow and nutrients to the injured area. Once the acute inflammatory response has resolved, pool therapy can be progressed. ROM exercises in conjunction with submaximal isometric strengthening exercises are performed initially for elbow flexor/extensor, wrist flexor, extensor, pronator, and supinator muscle groups. Rhythmic stabilization drills (partner assisted) for the aforementioned muscles groups can be initiated to enhance proprioceptive feedback and neuromuscular control.

Phase 2—Enhanced Mobility/ Intermediate Phase

Phase 2 is initiated when the patient is able to demonstrate full ROM and exhibit minimal pain/tenderness to the elbow, wrist, and hand. The goals of this phase of aquatic rehabilitation are to further enhance elbow, wrist, and hand mobility; gradually rebuild strength/endurance; and regain neuromuscular control of the upper extremity. Stretching exercises are implemented to maintain and progress ROM at the elbow, forearm, and hand. Elbow extension and forearm pronation are particularly important to the overhead athlete. The use of paddles/wands can be implemented to further enhance strengthening to elbow extensors and forearm pronators by increasing the resistance to flow. Strengthening exercises are progressed to incorporate isotonic strengthening of the elbow, wrist, and hand using body weight and/or hand paddles along with neuromuscular control exercises D2 PNF patterns (Figure 5-13), which

are "spiral and diagonal" in character and combine motion in all 3 planes: flexion/extension, abduction/adduction, and transverse rotation for upper extremity activation, and wrist flips integrate functional muscle firing patterns similar to demands faced in athletics, work environments, and general activities of daily living. These exercises should be performed in deeper water to challenge the patient to maintain proper trunk and pelvic stabilization while performing upper extremity movement patterns. Appropriate considerations should be applied to patients who demonstrate difficulty maintaining upright positions when performing exercises in deeper water. Supervision may or may not be necessary based on the skill level of the patient.

Phase 3—Advanced Strengthening Phase

Phase 3 prepares the patient for activities encountered in his or her environment. The goals of this phase are to increase strength, endurance, and neuromuscular control in order to return the patient to sport, work, or general activity. Principles of land-based therapy can be applied to incorporate interval sport programs in conjunction with aquatic rehabilitation. Work-hardening/conditioning programs, interval sport programs, and task-simulated aquatic movement patterns are performed to challenge the patient to meet the demands of his or her field, preferably in deeper water. Sport-specific tennis movements such as forehands and backhands may be performed in deeper water (Figure 5-14). Simulation of the golf swing can also be implemented in this stage. The principles of flow and buoyancy will challenge the patient to maintain stability throughout the lumbopelvic complex in order to perform the movement.

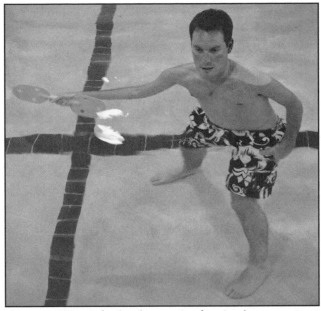

Figure 5-14. Tennis forehand promoting functional movement patterns. (Reprinted with permission from Leonard C. Macrina, MSPT, SCS, CSCS.)

This exercise can be progressed by adding a fin or hand paddle to increase resistance throughout the total arc of motion (Figure 5-15). Patients should exhibit full ROM; exhibit 4/5 strength of the elbow, wrist, and hand upon manual muscle testing; demonstrate satisfactory clinical exam; and exhibit no pain or tenderness upon palpation of elbow, wrist, and hand structures prior to advancement from this phase.

Phase 4—Return to Activity Phase

The final phase of elbow, wrist, and hand aquatic rehabilitation is returning to work, athletics, or activities of daily living. Movement patterns that are task related can be performed in shallow water to help adapt to the force of gravity. The patient is to continue flexibility, strength, endurance, and neuromuscular control exercises to maintain alignment of collagen, joint ROM, nourishment to articular cartilage, proprioceptive feedback to capsular structures, and maintenance of tissue homeostasis.

Conclusion

Aquatic therapy provides an exceptional environment for the rehabilitation of patients with shoulder, elbow, wrist, and hand impairments; functional limitations; and disabilities. Rehabilitation focuses on restoration of ROM, increased mobility, advancement of strength, and establishment of functional neuromuscular firing patterns to return a patient to work, athletics, or activities of daily living safely. Whether postinjury or postsurgical, aquatic therapy of the shoulder, elbow, wrist, and hand should follow a progressive multiphase approach in order to promote

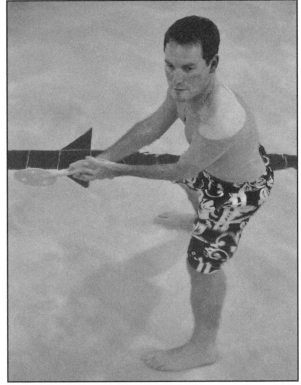

Figure 5-15. Golf swing utilized with resistance from the water to enhance the patient's dynamic movement patterns. (Reprinted with permission from Leonard C. Macrina, MSPT, SCS, CSCS.)

homeostatic conditions to healing tissues. Initiation of aquatic therapy will depend on the severity of the injury, inflammation/effusion associated with the injury, communication between the physician and rehabilitation specialist. The clinician should have a good understanding of the differences between land- and water-based programs in order to successfully progress the patient in a safe and concise manner.

The aforementioned physical properties of water, in conjunction with the physiologic effects at the cellular/tissue level with exercise of an immersed object, demonstrate the importance of using water as a medium for healing.

References

1. Cole AJ, Becker BE. *Comprehensive Aquatic Therapy.* 2nd ed. Philadelphia: Butterworth Heinemann; 2004.
2. Ruoti RG, Morris DM, Cole AJ. *Aquatic Rehabilitation.* Philadelphia: Lippincott-Raven Publishers; 1997.
3. Speer KP, Cavanaugh JT, Warren RF, Day L, Wickiewicz TL. A role for hydrotherapy in shoulder rehabilitation. *Am J Sports Med.* 1993;21:850–853.
4. Becker BE. Aquatic therapy: scientific foundations and clinical rehabilitation applications. *PM R.* 2009;1:859–872.
5. Brady B, Redfern J, MacDougal G, Williams J. The addition of aquatic therapy to rehabilitation following surgical rotator cuff repair: a feasibility study. *Physiother Res Int.* 2008;13(3):153–161.
6. Prins J, Cutner D. Aquatic therapy in the rehabilitation of athletic injuries. *Clin Sports Med.* 1999;18:447–461.
7. Thein JM, Brody LT. Aquatic-based rehabilitation and training for the elite athlete. *J Orthop Sports Phys Ther.* 1998;27(1):32–41.

8. Thein JM, Brody LT. Aquatic-based rehabilitation and training for the shoulder. *J Athl Train.* 2000;35:382–389.

9. Warren CG, Lehmann JF, Koblanski JN. Heat and stretch procedures: an evaluation using rat tail tendon. *Arch Phys Med Rehabil.* 1976;57(3):122–126.

10. Ciolek JJ. Cryotherapy. Review of physiological effects and clinical application. *Cleve Clin Q.* 1985;52:193–201.

11. Fujisawa H, Suenaga N, Minami A. Electromyographic study during isometric exercise of the shoulder in head-out water immersion. *J Shoulder Elbow Surg.* 1998;7:491–494.

12. Kelly BT, Roskin LA, Kirkendall DT, Speer KP. Shoulder muscle activation during aquatic and dry land exercises in nonimpaired subjects. *J Orthop Sports Phys Ther.* 2000;30:204–210.

13. Nuber GW, Jobe FW, Perry J, Moynes DR, Antonelli D. Fine wire electromyography analysis of muscles of the shoulder during swimming. *Am J Sports Med.* 1986;14:7–11.

14. Apreleva M, Hasselman CT, Debski RE, Fu FH, Woo SL, Warner JJ. A dynamic analysis of glenohumeral motion after simulated capsulolabral injury. A cadaver model. *J Bone Joint Surg Am.* 1998;80:474–480.

15. Cain PR, Mutschler TA, Fu FH, Lee SK. Anterior stability of the glenohumeral joint. A dynamic model. *Am J Sports Med.* 1987;15:144–148.

16. Harryman DT II, Sidles JA, Clark JM, McQuade KJ, Gibb TD, Matsen FA III. Translation of the humeral head on the glenoid with passive glenohumeral motion. *J Bone Joint Surg Am.* 1990;72:1334–1343.

17. Saha AK. Dynamic stability of the glenohumeral joint. *Acta Orthop Scand.* 1971;42(6):491–505.

18. Wilk KE, Arrigo CA, Andrews JR. Current concepts: the stabilizing structures of the glenohumeral joint. *J Orthop Sports Phys Ther.* 1997;25(6):364–379.

19. Reinold MM, Macrina LC, Wilk KE, et al. Electromyographic analysis of the supraspinatus and deltoid muscles during 3 common rehabilitation exercises. *J Athl Train.* 2007;42:464–469.

20. Reinold MM, Wilk KE, Fleisig GS, et al. Electromyographic analysis of the rotator cuff and deltoid musculature during common shoulder external rotation exercises. *J Orthop Sports Phys Ther.* 2004;34:385–394.

21. Lee SB, Kim KJ, O'Driscoll SW, Morrey BF, An KN. Dynamic glenohumeral stability provided by the rotator cuff muscles in the mid-range and end-range of motion. A study in cadavera. *J Bone Joint Surg Am.* 2000;82:849–857.

22. Burke WS, Vangsness CT, Powers CM. Strengthening the supraspinatus: a clinical and biomechanical review. *Clin Orthop Relat Res.* 2002(402):292–298.

23. Hughes RE, An KN. Force analysis of rotator cuff muscles. *Clin Orthop Relat Res.* 1996(330):75–83.

24. Liu J, Hughes RE, Smutz WP, Niebur G, Nan-An K. Roles of deltoid and rotator cuff muscles in shoulder elevation. *Clin Biomech (Bristol, Avon).* 1997;12:32–38.

25. Otis JC, Jiang CC, Wickiewicz TL, Peterson MG, Warren RF, Santner TJ. Changes in the moment arms of the rotator cuff and deltoid muscles with abduction and rotation. *J Bone Joint Surg Am.* 1994;76:667–676.

26. Rockwood CA, Matsen FA, Wirth MA, Harryman DT. *The Shoulder.* 2nd ed. Philadelphia: Saunders; 1998.

27. Sharkey NA, Marder RA. The rotator cuff opposes superior translation of the humeral head. *Am J Sports Med.* 1995;23(3):270–275.

28. Wilk KE, Arrigo C. Current concepts in the rehabilitation of the athletic shoulder. *J Orthop Sports Phys Ther.* 1993;18(1):365–378.

29. Wilk KE, Macrina LC, Reinold MM. Non-operative rehabilitation for traumatic and atraumatic glenohumeral instability. *N Am J Sports Phys Ther.* 2006;1:16–31.

30. Boushel R, Langberg H, Green S, Skovgaard D, Bulow J, Kjaer M. Blood flow and oxygenation in peritendinous tissue and calf muscle during dynamic exercise in humans. *J Physiol.* 2000;524(pt 1):305–313.

31. Hall CM, Brody LT. *Therapeutic Exercise: Moving Toward Function.* 2nd ed. Philadelphia: Lippincott Williams & Wilkins; 2005.

32. Brossmann J, Preidler KW, Pedowitz RA, White LM, Trudell D, Resnick D. Shoulder impingement syndrome: influence of shoulder position on rotator cuff impingement—an anatomic study. *Am J Roentgenol.* 1996;167:1511–1515.

33. Graichen H, Bonel H, Stammberger T, Englmeier KH, Reiser M, Eckstein F. Subacromial space width changes during abduction and rotation—a 3-D MR imaging study. *Surg Radiol Anat.* 1999;21:59–64.

34. Townsend H, Jobe FW, Pink M, Perry J. Electromyographic analysis of the glenohumeral muscles during a baseball rehabilitation program. *Am J Sports Med.* 1991;19(3):264–272.

35. Juul-Kristensen B, Bojsen-Moller F, Finsen L, et al. Muscle sizes and moment arms of rotator cuff muscles determined by magnetic resonance imaging. *Cells Tissues Organs.* 2000;167:214–222.

36. Juul-Kristensen B, Bojsen-Moller F, Holst E, Ekdahl C. Comparison of muscle sizes and moment arms of two rotator cuff muscles measured by ultrasonography and magnetic resonance imaging. *Eur J Ultrasound.* 2000;11:161–173.

37. Lephart SM, Henry TJ. The physiological basis for open and closed kinetic chain rehabilitation for the upper extremity. *J Sports Rehabil.* 1996;5:71–87.

38. Padua DA, Guskiewicz KM, Myers JB. Effects of closed kinetic chain, open kinetic chain and proprioceptive neuromuscular facilitation training on the shoulder. *J Athl Train.* 1999;34(suppl):83.

39. Wilk KE, Arrigo CA, Andrews JR. Closed and open kinetic chain exercises for the upper extremity. *J Sports Rehabil.* 1996;5:88–102.

40. Lephart SM, Pincivero DM, Giraldo JL, Fu FH. The role of proprioception in the management and rehabilitation of athletic injuries. *Am J Sports Med.* 1997;25:130–137.

41. Lephart SM, Riemann BL, Fu FH. Introduction to the sensorimotor system. In: Lephart SM, Fu FH, eds. *Proprioception and Neuromuscular Control in Joint Stability.* Champaign, Ill: Human Kinetics; 2000:16–26.

42. Frostick SP, Mohammad M, Ritchie DA. Sport injuries of the elbow. *Br J Sports Med.* 1999;33:301–311.

43. Safran MR. Elbow injuries in athletes. A review. *Clin Orthop Relat Res.* 1995(310):257–277.

44. Tullos HS, King JW. Throwing mechanism in sports. *Orthop Clin North Am.* 1973;4:709–720.

45. Wilk KE, Azar FM, Andrews JR. Conservative and operative rehabilitation of the elbow in sports. *Sports Med Arthrosc Rev.* 1995;3:237–258.

46. Wilk KE, Reinold MM, Andrews JR. Rehabilitation of the thrower's elbow. *Tech Hand Up Extrem Surg.* 2003;7:197–216.

47. Jackson DW, Silvino N, Reiman P. Osteochondritis in the female gymnast's elbow. *Arthroscopy.* 1989;5:129–136.

48. Morris M, Jobe FW, Perry J, Pink M, Healy BS. Electromyographic analysis of elbow function in tennis players. *Am J Sports Med.* 1989;17:241–247.

49. Kibler WB. Clinical biomechanics of the elbow in tennis: implications for evaluation and diagnosis. *Med Sci Sports Exerc.* 1994;26:1203–1206.

50. Rettig AC. Epidemiology of hand and wrist injuries in sports. *Clin Sports Med.* 1998;17:401–406.

51. Barr AE, Barbe MF, Clark BD. Work-related musculoskeletal disorders of the hand and wrist: epidemiology, pathophysiology, and sensorimotor changes. *J Orthop Sports Phys Ther.* 2004;34:610–627.

52. Clarke MT, Lyall HA, Grant JW, Matthewson MH. The histopathology of de Quervain's disease. *J Hand Surg Br.* 1998;23:732–734.

53. Case and Demographic Characteristics for Work-related Injuries and Illnesses Involving Days Away From Work. Bureau of Labor Statistics Web site. http://www.bls.gov/iif/oshcdnew1999.htm#99Supplemental_Tables. Accessed February 2011.

54. Wilk KE, Reinold MM, Andrews JR. Rehabilitation of the thrower's elbow. *Sports Med Arthrosc Rev.* 2003;11:79–95.

Aquatic Rehabilitation for the Spine

Timothy DiFrancesco, PT, DPT, ATC, CSCS, AQx, CMT and Lisa Pataky, PT, DPT

Low back pain (LBP) is a widespread problem, with close to 85% of people reporting at least one incidence of low back pain at some point in their life. It is the most common cause of referral to physical therapy and one of the leading causes of disability.[1] Eighty-five percent to 90% of patients who have LBP will return to all activities in 8 to 10 weeks; however, the 10% to 15% who do not will require rehabilitation and possibly surgery in the future.[1,2] From a public health standpoint, chronic LBP requires long-term treatment and restricts the ability of patients to work, making it one of the largest drains on the health resources of advanced industrialized societies.[3] A 2004 study analyzed health care expenses in the United States. The analysis found that back pain cost over $90 billion, of which $26 billion was spent directly on treating the back pain.[4]

Guidelines for the management of nonspecific chronic LBP recommend supervised exercise therapy as a first-line treatment for the reduction of pain and disability.[5] Exercise has been shown to improve pain and function in patients with LBP and is considered an important part of a multifaceted approach to the treatment of LBP.[1] Rehabilitation and therapeutic exercise for the spine, though beneficial, can often be challenging in terms of selecting the proper exercises given the impairments identified. Some of the difficulty arises from the fact that, unlike the hip or knee, the spine is multisegmented. It is made up of 33 vertebrae, 25 segmental linkages, and 3 joints at each linkage, all surrounding the neurological system and its vascular supply.

Each segment is linked with ligaments, capsules, discs, and muscles, presenting multiple possibilities for nociceptive input and a plethora of diagnoses and treatments.

Due to the unique properties of water, aquatic therapy is a perfect medium for rehabilitation of the spine. The buoyancy of the water allows the spine to be unloaded and exercises to be initiated earlier than may be possible on land. The importance of strengthening and stabilization exercises for the treatment of back pain is widely accepted; however, with land-based exercises axial loading and compression on the spine are unavoidable and often painful.[6] With aquatic therapy, the amount of weight bearing and loading through the spine can easily be altered by changing the level of submersion of the individual.[6,7] This allows for earlier initiation of therapy than would be possible on land. The basic premise for prescribing aquatic exercises for LBP patients is that buoyancy will reduce spinal loads and hydrostatic pressure and the temperature of the water will assist with balance and pain control, respectively.[7] Accordingly, patients with LBP who find it difficult to perform land-based exercises may successfully perform aquatic exercises first and then progress to more functional land-based exercises after a period of time. By using the properties of water, a graded exercise program can be created to help improve each individual's impairments and return to normal levels of functioning. Aquatic exercise has been shown to decrease pain and improve strength, range of motion, and quality of life in individuals with LBP.[8]

Wilk KE, Joyner DM. *The Use of Aquatics in Orthopedic and Sports Medicine Rehabilitation and Physical Conditioning (pp 71-80).*

Table 6-1.

Influence of Motion on the Spine

Direction of Motion	Size of Canal and Foramen	Tension on Nerve Root	Movement of Disc	Pressure on Spine/Disc
Extension	Decreases size	Decreases	Posteriorly	Increases
Flexion	Increases size	Increases	Anteriorly	Increases (highest in sitting)
Rotation	Increases contralaterally, decreases ipsilaterally	Increases contralaterally, decreases ipsilaterally	Contralateral	Increases ipsilaterally, decreases contralaterally
Side bending	Increases on contralateral side, decreases on ipsilateral side	Increases on contralateral side, decreases on ipsilateral side	Contralateral	Increased ipsilaterally, decreases contralaterally

AQUATIC THERAPY INTERVENTION FOR LOW BACK PAIN

Supervised exercise therapy is recommended for the treatment of LBP, and aquatic therapy can provide the ideal environment in which to initiate exercises. Water exercises provide several benefits over traditional land-based ones, including earlier initiation of exercises for patients with high levels of pain, increased support in the presence of strength or proprioceptive deficits, exercising with decreased axial or shear forces on the spine, and decreased pain due in part to the ability of warm water to decrease muscle spasm and tightness.[2]

One of the greatest advantages of aquatic therapy for the treatment of back pain is the ability to begin earlier interventions than would be possible using traditional land-based exercises. It is widely accepted that bed rest is detrimental to patients with LBP because muscles can atrophy and further weaken during this time.[2] Additionally, the decreased activation of muscles results in slower healing time for the intervertebral discs due to the lack of fluid flow.[2] Due to the unloading effects that buoyancy provides, an earlier and more aggressive treatment protocol can occur with aquatic therapy and therefore better results may be seen with this type of intervention.[2,9] A systematic review showed that aquatic therapy is a safe and effective treatment modality for patients with chronic LBP. There are high compliance rates with this type of intervention and it has been found to increase functional and quality of life outcome assessments such as the Oswestry Low Back Pain Disability Questionnaire and SF-36.[1,2,8,9] Additionally, these patients have been shown to gain self-confidence and self-efficacy because they are able to initiate early therapy with decreased feelings of pain while exercising.[2]

THEORY BEHIND EXERCISE PRESCRIPTION

The spine assists with transferring weight and loading from the pelvis and lower extremities to the head, arms, and trunk, in addition to providing support to the head. Understanding the basic concepts in the biomechanics of the spine will help to clarify how specific activities can exacerbate or alleviate symptoms in lumbar spine pathologies (Table 6-1).

Before initiating any aquatic therapy program, a thorough history and physical examination should be performed on land to determine all impairments and which exercises will be of the most benefit to the patient. As with any other injury, determining the source of the pain is crucial, and examination above and below the involved joint should be performed as well. Additionally, identification of motions and actions that exacerbate or alleviate the pain or centralize/peripheralize symptoms will aid in the selection of appropriate therapeutic exercises. Panjabi identified 3 systems (passive, active, and neuromuscular) that contribute to the stabilization of the spine, all of which must be taken into account when considering treatment protocols for LBP.[10]

Porterfield and DeRosa described 3 musculofascial systems of the lumbopelvic region that contribute to lumbopelvic stability and mobility: the thoracolumbar fascia, the abdominal system, and the system of the hip/fascia lata.[11] These 3 systems function as shock absorbers to decrease the forces placed on the spine during daily and recreational activities. The muscles that help form the thoracolumbar fascia are critical to the rehabilitation of LBP, especially in those individuals with discogenic pain, because contraction of any of these muscles results in subsequent compression across the discs and promotion of synovial fluid. The muscles that are embedded within, intersect with, or are related to the thoracolumbar fascia include the gluteus maximus, latissimus dorsi, gluteus medius, external and internal obliques, transversus abdominus, erector spinae, quadratus lumborum, and multifidi. Appendix I describes a treatment protocol and lumbar exercises in the aquatic area.

Knowing that the thoracolumbar fascia is directly connected to the latissimus dorsi magnifies the importance of the connection between the gluteus maximus and the latissimus dorsi. Due to its attachment to the thoracolumbar fascia, contraction of the gluteus maximus alone will increase tension in the fascial systems and therefore increase lumbar stability. Furthermore, simultaneous contraction of the gluteus maximus and the contralateral latissimus dorsi creates even more tension in the thoracolumbar fascia and therefore greater lumbar stability.[11] Understanding these interconnections between musculofascial systems allows one to develop a more effective and efficient plan when treating or preventing low back pathology. When you combine that knowledge with an awareness of how the central nervous system and neural sequencing are related, you will have a powerful systematic approach on managing spine pathology.

In addition to choosing exercises that coincide with motions that alleviate symptoms (ie, standing or extension exercises with nerve root compression or sitting, flexion-based exercises for individuals with stenosis), aquatic exercise for this population should include exercises that improve and focus on trunk stabilization, proprioception, and dynamic control.[2] Exercises to improve the strength and endurance of trunk muscles are often included in fitness and rehabilitation programs because properly conditioned trunk muscles will reduce the risk of low back injuries during physical exertions and allow for arm and leg movements to be performed more forcefully and accurately.[7] Exercises should also focus on strengthening of proximal trunk muscles to promote proper posture and postural control to allow for efficient movements during all activities.[2]

As on land, exercises should begin with teaching the patient how to find a neutral spine and working on posterior pelvic tilts and activation of transversus abdominus (TA) and lumbar multifidi muscles. Exercises should then be progressed to activation of the TA while performing marching or alternative leg activities and activation of the multifidi while performing a bird dog activity. Once these have been mastered, and as pain decreases, exercises should further progress to activation of both of these muscles while performing more functional activities such as squats, lunges, lat pull-downs, walking, and running. Eventually, individuals should practice functional activities that mimic their daily lives; for example, manual laborers should practicing lifting, bending, and carrying with emphasis placed on proper technique and functional training. Furthermore,

athletes can work on sport-specific movements that may be too aggressive with land-based exercises and can participate in deep water or treadmill running (see Chapter 2, Figure 2-5) to maintain their cardiovascular fitness levels while away from their sport.[2]

Exercises should also begin at a deeper depth of water to more fully unload the spine. Deep water exercises allow the patient to move all joints through a full range of motion while eliminating loads to the spine. Additionally, buoyancy-assistive devices such as flotation belts can be worn to allow for full movement of the extremities.[2] Patients should also progress from deep water walking and running to more shallow water walking and running to simulate and prepare for return to land-based exercises with full loading through the spine.

Pool temperatures can range from 25°C to 40°C depending on the goal of the exercise and therapy session, with cooler temperatures being used for acute inflammation and some exercises and warmer temperatures being used for increasing blood and oxygen flow to muscles, decreasing muscle spasm, and assisting with pain relief.[2,6] Exercises should be performed 2 to 3 times per week and should begin with all aquatic-based therapy and then progress to land-based exercises as pain and function improve. Individuals participating in aquatic therapy 3 times a week should then progress to 2 days of aquatic and 1 day of land-based and then 1 day of aquatic and 2 days of land-based exercises until they are able to complete their entire exercise protocol using only land-based exercises.

ACUTE LOW BACK PAIN

Acute LBP can occur as a result of acute facet joint locking, muscle spasm, or strain or as the result of trauma. Individuals with acute back pain can often have higher pain levels, resulting in decreased ability to complete activities, especially weight-bearing ones, and higher incidence of bed rest. It is widely accepted now that bed rest is harmful to these individuals and that the sooner they can begin moving and initiating therapeutic exercises, the better their prognosis. Aquatic therapy can provide the perfect medium for this population to initiate early, pain-free exercises and activities.

With acute LBP the warm water can be used to reduce pain and allow patients to begin some exercises early on, because immobilization can be harmful.[2] Initiation of therapy in water could be a good starting point, with further progression to land as individuals are able to tolerate greater amounts of weight bearing. Usually, these individuals are in great pain and any increased forces through the spine are painful. These patients would therefore enjoy the buoyancy effect of aquatic therapy, which serves to decrease loads through the spine while still providing the opportunity to activate their muscles and work on dynamic stabilization of

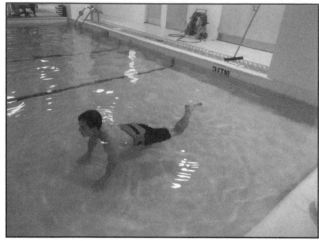

Figure 6-1. Quad extension.

the spine. However, because of the substantial reduction of electromyographic activity in water, a patient must progress toward land-based exercises to more fully activate the trunk muscles.[7]

FRACTURES, TRAUMA, AND SPONDYLOLYSIS

Acute LBP can occur not just from locking of the facet joint, which often can be treated with a couple treatments of lumbar manipulation and functional training, but from stress fractures, pars interarticularis fractures, and trauma to the spine. Stress fractures and spondylolysis (fracture of the pars interarticularis) result from overuse or traumatic injuries to the spine and are worse with motions that produce extension, hyperextension, and repeated shear forces. Avoidance of these motions should be taken into account when choosing appropriate therapeutic exercises. It is also important to remember that with active stress fractures or spinal fractures there will be interrupted communication between spinal musculature and the central nervous system, resulting in further susceptibility to destabilizing loads in the stressed or fractured segments. Exercises with a flexion bias, such as those in sitting, hook lying, or a bicycle position, should be utilized to allow for healing and decreased exacerbation of symptoms. Early exercises should focus on maintenance of neutral spine, pelvic tilts, and activation of dynamic spinal stabilizers such as the TA and multifidi. As pain decreases and function returns, exercise should progress as typical spine rehabilitation would, with a focus on strengthening of the glutes and latissimus dorsi, activation of spinal stabilizers in more functional positions, walking, and eventual return to running.

Motor sports, high-velocity sports, and collision sports are capable of producing significant forces to the cervical,

thoracic, and lumbar spine. Fractures, fracture dislocations, and dislocations can occur with and without neurologic injury. Blunt trauma may produce rib fractures and transverse process fractures. Any of the ligamentous structures may be injured, leading to very specific treatments. The treatment varies depending on the degree of trauma. After on-the-field management and transfer to a care facility, further treatment plans can be made depending on exam and imaging. Some traumatic injuries can be managed conservatively, but surgical intervention may be required. The procedure will be determined by the injury. Possibilities include bracing, rigid bracing (HALO), and surgical fusions of various types. Depending on the amount of neurological involvement in a diagnosis of this nature, the pool may not only be appropriate but necessary. The aquatic medium provides an environment in which an individual with significant neurological impairment can walk and receive resistance during movement in all planes simply while performing basic gait training. All core stabilization, activation, and strengthening is appropriate when the doctor lifts precautions.

Compression fractures are another type of injury that result in acute LBP and are often a result of osteopenia or osteoporosis combined with a fall or traumatic injury. These fractures sometimes require surgical intervention and treatment protocols, and progression will be based on whether or not the patient can be managed in a purely conservative manner. The fact that the patient has suffered a compression fracture typically indicates that there is decreased stability of the spine and therefore spinal stabilization should be the major focus of exercises for this population. Exercises for spinal stabilization should focus on mid-range exercises with the spine in neutral and cocontraction of all core muscles to provide dynamic stabilization.[2] Modified swimming can also be used to promote trunk stabilization and core activation. The aquatic environment is a very safe place to begin functional treatment with this diagnosis due to the fact that it creates a buoyant pressure relief on the compressed boney tissue. Ultimately this patient will require weight-bearing and aggressive core stabilization activities, but the water provides a head start in this process during early rehab when the patient would otherwise be unable to tolerate land-based functional rehabilitation.

Exercises for patients with compression fractures include the following:

- Early phase: quadruped belly breathing, quadruped glute extension, quadruped glute abduction with extension, hip extension, abduction and adduction with a noodle, pelvic tilts, abdominal hallowing (Figures 6-1 to 6-5)
- Intermediate phase: squats, lunges, bicycle kicks, marching, water walking, rotation with tubing, lat pull-downs with tubing or resistance of water using

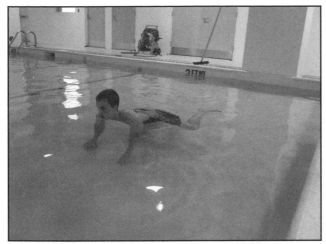

Figure 6-2. Quad abduction.

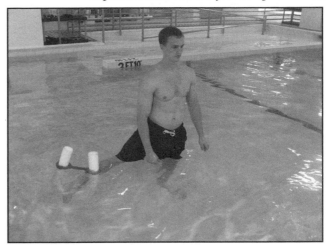

Figure 6-3. Hip abduction.

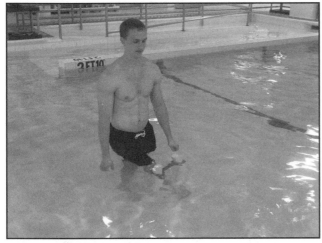

Figure 6-4. Hip adduction.

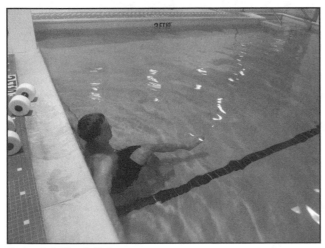

Figure 6-6. Bicycle kicks.

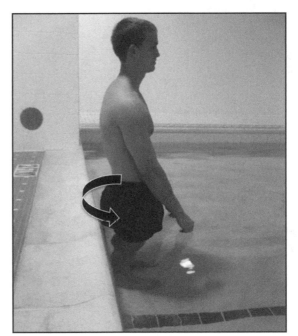

Figure 6-5. Pelvic tilts.

SPONDYLOLISTHESIS

Spondylolisthesis occurs when one vertebra slips out of position in relation to the segments above and below. This most commonly occurs in the lumbar spine, in particular at the L5/S1 segment. Though spondylolisthesis can be a stable or unstable diagnosis, extreme end ranges of motions should still be avoided, because these will most likely be painful for this patient population. The buoyant environment of the water is a prime place to initiate isometric core stabilization and strengthening activities. Rehabilitation for this diagnosis is quite similar to that of stress fractures and spondylolysis and includes most of the same exercises.

Exercises for this population include the following:

- Early phase: quadruped belly breathing, quadruped glute extension, quadruped glute abduction with

paddles, planks and side planks, bird dog (Figures 6-6 to 6-9)

- Later phase: step-ups, step-downs, lunges and squats with weights or medicine ball, dead lifts, dumbbell swings, water running (Figures 6-10 to 6-13)

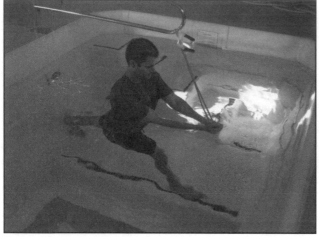

Figure 6-7. Core antirotation press.

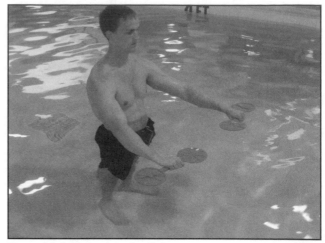

Figure 6-8. Latissimus dorsi pull-down.

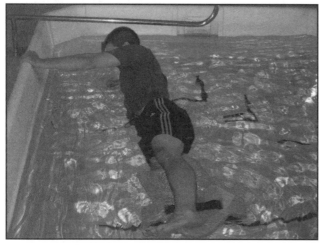

Figure 6-9. Side plank.

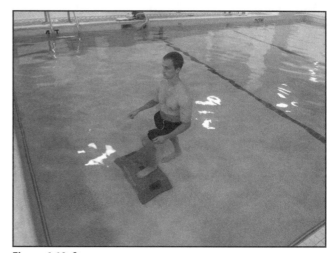

Figure 6-10. Step ups.

extension, hip extension, abduction and adduction with a noodle, pelvic tilts, abdominal hallowing (see Figures 6-1 to 6-5)

- Intermediate phase: squats, lunges, bicycle kicks, marching, water walking, rotation with tubing, lat pull-downs with tubing or resistance of water using paddles, planks and side planks, bird dog (see Figures 6-6 to 6-9)

- Later phase: step-ups, step-downs, lunges and squats with weights or medicine ball, dead lifts, dumbbell swings, water running (see Figures 6-10 to 6-13)

DISCOGENIC DISEASE AND NERVE ROOT COMPRESSION

LBP can also occur from disc disease and nerve root compression. With repeated flexion and degeneration of the disc, the disc begins to migrate and protrude posteriorly, which can result in compression on the spinal nerves resulting in radicular symptoms. Patients with this diagnosis often complain not only of back pain but buttock, thigh, and lower leg pain as well. Typically these individuals will have relief with standing or lying down and exacerbation of symptoms with sitting or any action involving forward flexion. Therefore, exercises should take place in a supine, standing, or extension-biased position and sitting and bicycle positions should be avoided. Aquatic therapy is an ideal environment for this population as well because they often have very high levels of pain and sometimes cannot complete any weight-bearing activities. Patients with severe nerve root compression may have to start with horizontal exercises (supine and prone) and then move to standing; however, due to the decreased weight bearing and axial loading that the water provides, they may be able to start standing and weight-bearing exercises sooner than they would be able to on land.[2] Traction is also beneficial for this population and can be achieved by adding weights to their ankles or waist to get distraction to the spine and decreased pressure on the disc.[2]

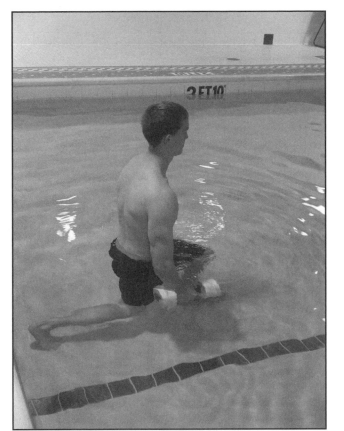

Figure 6-11. Lunge with weight.

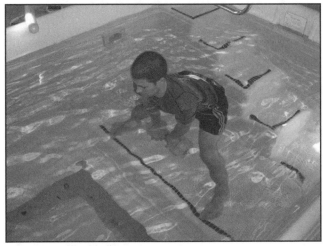

Figure 6-13. Dumbbell swing.

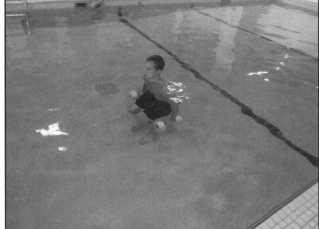

Figure 6-12. Squat with weight.

awareness to help reduce and even eliminate pressure on the disc. Functional training on how to complete activities while avoiding repeated flexion should be the focus of therapy as well. Though aquatic therapy is an ideal and safe early intervention for this population, manual therapy on land may often need to be performed concomitantly to achieve optimal results.

Exercises for this population include the following:

- Early phase: pelvic tilts, activation of TA and multifidi in supine or quadruped, lat pull-downs using water's resistance and paddles or exercise bands, extension in standing, bridging (see Figures 6-5, 6-8, and 6-14)

- Intermediate phase: squats, lunges, bird dog, planks, side planks, TA activation with marching or alternating leg kicks, core antirotation press (CARP) with tubing, hip extension, abduction and adduction with noodle, walking (see Figures 6-3, 6-4, 6-6, 6-7, 6-18, and 6-19)

- Late phase: overhead squat with weight or noodle, dead lifts, dumbbell swings, running, step-ups, step-downs (see Figures 6-10 to 6-13)

SPINAL STENOSIS AND DEGENERATION

Spinal stenosis occurs as a result of a narrowing of the intervertebral foramen and can be degenerative or congenital in nature. As the narrowing progresses, impingement on nerves can occur, resulting in neurological symptoms into the buttock, thigh, and lower leg. As mentioned earlier, flexion serves to open the joint spaces and foramina, whereas extension and ipsilateral side bend and rotation further close down the openings. Therefore, with this population, exercises should focus on flexion-biased positions such as hook lying, sitting, and bicycle position. Though surgery is sometimes indicated for the treatment of this pathology,

Disc herniations should be treated conservatively for at least 6 weeks before surgery is even considered. Extension-oriented exercises have been shown to be effective for this population and oftentimes surgery can be avoided.[12] Exercises that activate the muscles associated with the thoracolumbar fascia should be incorporated because they result in intermittent compression along the spine, providing increased fluid flow to the discs to aid in healing and reabsorption. In addition to exercises that place the spine in an extended position, patients should be educated on how to maintain a neutral or extended spine as well as postural

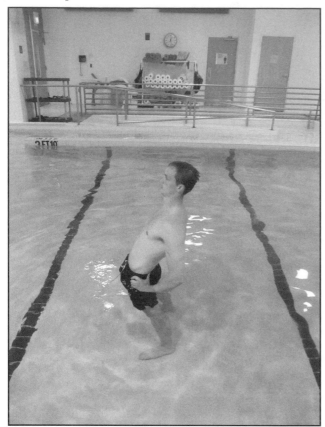

Figure 6-14. Extension in standing.

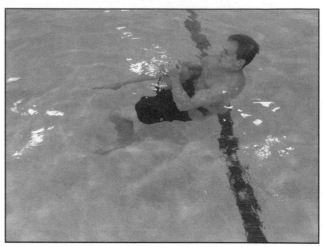

Figure 6-15. Knees to chest.

conservative intervention for at least 6 weeks is still recommended for the initial intervention, and Whitman et al had successful results with therapeutic exercises for this population.[13] Though the narrowing of the canal cannot be reversed without surgical intervention, exercises that focus on increasing hip extension, spinal stabilization, and core strengthening can assist with reduced symptoms and increased function. Additionally, activation of the muscles associated with the thoracolumbar fascia, such as gluteus maximus and latissimus dorsi, can assist in achieving intermittent compression along the spine, which can help with healing of the involved structures. Flexibility exercises for the hip flexors, hamstrings, and gastroc/soleus complex should be included as well because individuals with spinal stenosis tend to sit for prolonged periods of time because they feel more relief in this position. Though aquatic therapy is an ideal and safe early intervention for this population, manual therapy on land may often need to be performed concomitantly to achieve optimal results.

Exercises for this population include the following:

- Early phase: TA and multifidi activation, posterior pelvic tilts, knees to chest, quadruped extension and abduction, hip flexor/hamstring/gastrocnemius stretches (see Figures 6-1, 6-2, 6-5, and 6-15 to 6-18)

- Intermediate phase: squats, lunges, CARP with tubing, hip extension, abduction and adduction with noodle, lat pull-downs with water resistance and paddles or tubing, bird dog, planks, side planks, hook lying marching or alternating leg kicks, bridging, walking (see Figures 6-3, 6-4, and 6-6 to 6-9)

- Late phase: lunge and squat with weights, dead lifts, step-ups, dumbbell swing, running (see Figures 6-1 and 6-10 to 6-13)

LOW BACK PAIN AND PREGNANCY

Between 50% and 70% of expectant women suffer from pregnancy-related back and pelvic girdle pain, leading to one of the most common reasons for lost work time, early initiation of maternity leave, and decreased ability to perform activities of daily living, instrumental activities of daily living, and recreational activities.[1,14] Causes are thought to be related to loosening of the pelvic ligaments as the body prepares for childbirth, and recommended treatments include exercise therapy, back support, massage, and education.[1] A recent systematic review by Stuge et al on exercise in the treatment of pregnancy-related back and pelvic girdle pain concluded that exercise is beneficial but not necessarily superior to other interventions.[15]

Though exercise is accepted as a safe and effective treatment for pregnant women suffering from back pain, the spinal loads that occur with weight-bearing exercises often result in increased levels of pain. The water provides a safe environment for pregnant women because the warm water provides pain-relieving effects and the buoyancy serves to reduce loading on the back and pelvic girdle. Additionally, the buoyancy and hydrostatic pressure of water assist in supporting the spine and pelvis.[1] A systematic review revealed reduced number of sick days related to LBP and decreased pain on the Visual Analog Scale in pregnant women after aquatic therapy.[1] Pregnant women who undertook a 1-hour active aquatic session once a week had significantly less

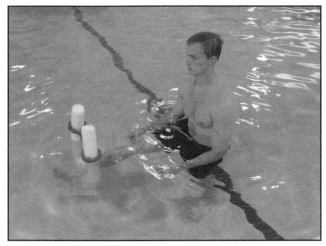

Figure 6-16. Hamstring stretch.

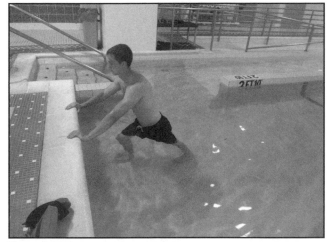

Figure 6-17. Gastrocnemius stretch.

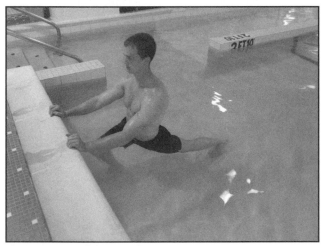

Figure 6-18. Hip flexor stretch.

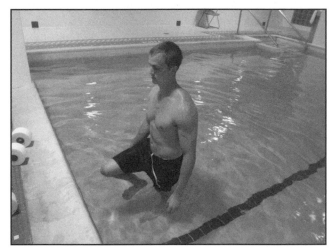

Figure 6-19. Standing marching.

pregnancy-related back and pelvic pain and were 34% less often absent from work than pregnant women who received normal prenatal care.[1,15]

Exercises for this population should focus mostly on dynamic stabilization of the spine as well as general aerobic exercise and core strengthening and should be chosen and adjusted based on tolerance and how far along in the pregnancy the patient is.

Exercises for this population include the following: TA and multifidi activation in whatever position is most comfortable; bird dog; supine, hook lying, or standing marching; squats; lunges; lat pull-downs with the water and paddles for resistance or with tubing; hip extension; abduction and adduction with noodles; walking and running; planks (see Figures 6-3, 6-4, 6-8, 6-9, and 6-19).

CONCLUSION

Exercise is widely recognized as an ideal intervention for individuals with back pain or spinal pathologies. Though early initiation of rehabilitation is key, weight-bearing exercises on land often place too much stress along the spine and result in increased pain and decreased function. Aquatic therapy allows these individuals to begin exercising earlier by using the unique properties of water to unload but stabilize the spine, allowing for pain-free exercise. Aquatic therapy also aids in breaking the pain cycle, allowing these individuals to become more mobile and progress to traditional land-based exercises earlier. Aquatic therapy should not be used in isolation but should be used as a starting point for this population. Patients should begin with aquatic therapy and slowly progress to incorporating more land-based exercises until they are able to successfully complete a pain-free exercise regimen on land. Patients should also be reassessed frequently to determine how well they are progressing and determine the appropriate time to initiate land-based therapy. This chapter should serve as a starting point for an exercise program for spine pathologies because these often require highly specialized guidance and a team approach that includes close communication among all members of the rehabilitation team in order to assist with maximum recovery for the patient.

REFERENCES

1. Waller B, Lambeck J, Daly D. Therapeutic aquatic exercise in the treatment of low back pain: a systematic review. *Clin Rehabil.* 2009;23:3–14.

2. Konlian C. Aquatic therapy: making a wave in the treatment of low back injuries. *Orthop Nurs.* 1999;18:11–20.

3. Constant F, Guillemin F, Collin JF, Boulangé M. Use of spa therapy to improve the quality of life of chronic low back pain patients. *Med Care.* 1998;36:1309–1314.

4. Luo X, Pietrobon R, Sun SX, et al. Estimates and patterns of direct health care expenditures among individuals with back pain in the United States. *Spine.* 2004;29:79–86.

5. Cuesta-Vargas AI, Heywood S. Aerobic fitness testing in chronic nonspecific low back pain: a comparison of deep-water running and cycle ergometry. *Am J Phys Med Rehabil.* 2011;90:1030–1035.

6. Ariyoshi M, Sonoda K, Nagata K, et al. Efficacy of aquatic exercise for patients with low-back pain. *Kurume Med J.* 1999;46(2):91–96.

7. Bressel E, Doiny DG, Gibbons M. Trunk muscle activity during exercises performed on land and in water. *Med Sci Sports Exerc.* 2011;43:1927–1932.

8. McIlveen B, Robertson VJ. A randomized controlled study of the outcome of hydrotherapy for subjects with low back or back and leg pain. *Physiotherapy.* 1998;84:17–26.

9. Dundar U, Solak O, Yigit I, Evcik D, Kavuncu V. Clinical effectiveness of aquatic exercise to treat chronic low back pain: a randomized controlled trial. *Spine.* 2009;34:1436–1440.

10. Panjabi MM. The stabilizing system of the spine. Part I. Function, dysfunction, adaptation, and enhancement. *J Spinal Disord.* 1992;5:383–389.

11. Porterfield JA, DeRosa C. *Mechanical Low Back Pain: Perspectives in Functional Anatomy.* 2nd ed. Philadelphia: Saunders; 1998.

12. Browder DA, Childs JD, Cleland JA, Fritz JM. Effectiveness of an extension-oriented treatment approach in a subgroup of subjects with low back pain: a randomized clinical trial. *Phys Ther.* 2007;87:1608–1618.

13. Whitman JM, Flynn TW, Childs JD, et al. A comparison between two physical therapy treatment programs for patients with lumbar spinal stenosis: a randomized clinical trial. *Spine.* 2006;31:2541–2549.

14. Kihlstrand M, Stenman B, Nilsson S, Axelsson O. Water-gymnastics reduced the intensity of back/low back pain in pregnant women. *Acta Obstet Gynecol Scand.* 1999;78:180–185.

15. Stuge B, Hilde G, Vøllestad N. Physical therapy for pregnancy-related low back and pelvic pain: a systematic review. *Acta Obstet Gynecol Scand.* 2003;82:983–990.

7

Chronic Pain
Fibromyalgia and Other Syndromes

Daniel Seidler, PT, MS

Fibromyalgia (FM) is a chronic pain syndrome characterized by widespread nonarticular pain, stiffness, multiple tender points, and fatigue.[1] Other common symptoms include diminished pain threshold, sleep disturbance, fatigue, headaches, morning stiffness, parasthesias, and anxiety. Nonrestorative sleep is common in FM, with about 75% of patients reporting sleep disturbances, including early, middle, or late insomnia; hypersomnia; and frequent awakening.[2] The organic nature of the abnormal central pain processing in FM has been demonstrated in many studies.[3]

Patients report that symptoms have a severe impact on their function in everyday life, including such basic activities as walking and upper extremity activities of daily living (ADL).[4,5] Patients' muscular performance is often found to be impaired.[6-9]

Initially called *fibrositis*, the name was changed to FM when it became evident that inflammation was not part of this condition.[10] The prevalence of FM is reported to be 3.4% in women and 0.5% in men, affecting women 7 to 10 times more than men.[11] Demographic and social characteristics associated with the presence of FM are Western culture, female gender, failing to complete high school, low-income status, and depression.[1,2]

The etiology and pathogenesis of FM remain relatively unknown. In different patients, FM has had differing origins. Some patients report having had FM symptoms since childhood. Others slowly develop FM in adulthood or become afflicted with FM following a traumatic or stressful incident. Patients have also reported waking one morning with flu-like aches but never getting ill, just staying in pain.

Commonly, there is an association with childhood stress or prolonged or severe stress.

There is no specific, objective clinical diagnostic test for FM, but many pathophysiological indicators are typically present in patients with FM:

- Increased levels of substance P (the agent that signals the brain to register pain) in the cerebrospinal fluid
- Neuroendocrine disruption
- Polymodal sensitivity
- Sympathetic hyperactivity
- Abnormal brain involvement

Are FM patients genetically predisposed to the condition? Are the physiological changes a result of physical feedback from the neurological system? Cause and effect have not been definitively determined as of yet. All indications suggest that some individuals are born with a predisposition for FM. Their experiences and lifestyle likely trigger and worsen the condition in varying degrees.

Regardless of which came first, it is evident that patients with FM are hypersensitive to external stimuli. Sheets rubbing on their skin or clothes of certain material can be unbearable. Joints often feel swollen or inflamed when there is scant objective evidence of irregularity. The neurophysiological abnormalities that exist provide an explanation. As explained by Dr. Michael Gilewski, a neuropsychologist at Cedars-Sinai Medical Center, in the documentary *Living With Fibromyalgia: A Journey of Hope and Understanding*: "the body and brain of the patient with FM are out of balance."[12]

Wilk KE, Joyner DM. *The Use of Aquatics in Orthopedic and Sports Medicine Rehabilitation and Physical Conditioning (pp 81-89).*

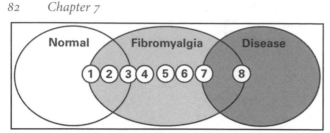

Figure 7-1. The FM spectrum. (Reprinted with permission from Mark J. Pellegrino, MD.)

FM has been classified as a central sensitivity syndrome, a condition of general overreactivity of the central nervous system (CNS) to a wide spectrum of stimulation.[2] The body experiences something and the CNS processes it differently than it would in a person without FM. FM and related disorders appear to reflect deficiencies in serotonergic and noradrenergic, but not opioidergic, transmission in the CNS. A research team led by Laurence Bradley at the University of Alabama at Birmingham has used single-photon emission computed tomography scans to demonstrate the apparent low levels of regional cerebral blood flow, which helps regulate the transmission of brain signals within the CNS, in the brain structures of FM patients.[13] Investigators continue to study the brain neurotransmitter substance P, which exists in increased amounts in FM patients—in fact, 3 times more than in normal controls.[14] Of continued interest is why the neurotransmitter serotonin (which modifies the intensity of pain signals entering the brain) appears to be deficient in patients with FM. In fact, many of the medications currently used to treat FM work to counteract this deficit. The results of these chemical changes are allodynia (painful responses to nonpainful stimuli) and hyperalgesia (heightened responses to painful stimuli) in FM patients.

Do the biochemical changes in the patient with FM lead to his or her symptoms or do the symptoms lead to these changes? It is possible that both processes occur simultaneously and that they amplify each other. FM pain causes changes in the CNS and those changes lead to additional changes in perception. Treatments that run counter to this process appear to effectively reverse the course of FM.

THE FIBROMYALGIA SPECTRUM

In his book, *Fibromyalgia: Up Close and Personal*, Dr. Mark Pellegrino outlined a FM spectrum (Figure 7-1).[15] The 8 stages he defined are as follows:

1. Predisposed state: Asymptomatic, no clinical signs of FM, hereditary factors present.

2. Prodromal (preceding) state: No widespread pain, pain at times and possibly headaches, fatigue, or irritable bowel syndrome.

3. Undiagnosed FM: Mild, chronic pain; may or may not meet the American College of Rheumatology (ACR) criteria of 11 of 18.

4. Regional FM: Very similar to myofascial pain syndrome (arguably synonymous); trigger points, tender points, shortened ropy muscles, adenosine triphosphate abnormalities, sympathetic nerve dysfunction, peripheral and central mechanisms; early treatment helps to prevent progression.

5. Generalized FM: Widespread pain and tender points, usually meeting the ACR criteria.

6. FM with particular associated conditions: FM has led to other conditions that need to be addressed in addition to the FM.

7. FM with coexisting mild disease: Other diseases exist concurrently with FM, but do not necessarily cause it; FM will worsen as the disease does; these diseases can be hormonal, infectious, rheumatic, arthritic, neurological, and lung conditions.

8. Secondary FM reactive to disease: In these cases, FM has developed as a result of a disease.

Whether they were born with the condition, are predisposed to it, or acquired FM from the external environment, patients with FM are often misdiagnosed, misunderstood, or stigmatized. It is not uncommon for them to see several physicians in search of an appropriate diagnosis. They may try an array of pharmacological options, attempt several types of therapy, and ultimately hop around the medical community in search of answers and solutions. They may have other conditions that can complicate the diagnosis of FM. Other musculoskeletal, neurological, or endocrine syndromes can overlap FM symptoms and confuse the diagnosis and treatment process.

DIAGNOSIS

Historically, FM has been diagnosed by the existence of the ACR criteria: concurrent presence of widespread pain on both sides of the body, above and below the waist for at least 3 months, and tenderness on palpation in at least 11 of 18 tender point sights (Figure 7-2). No exclusions are made for the presence of concomitant radiographic or laboratory abnormalities. An adequate assessment for FM requires that the practitioner systematically palpate the 18 sites. A moderate and consistent degree of pressure should be used in digital palpation (using the thumb of the dominant hand) of these tender points. The amount of force applied should be 8.8 lb (4.0 kg), which should blanch the examiner's thumbnail.[3,16-18]

FM will often overlap with other diagnoses. Because it is a diagnosis of inclusion, if the ACR criteria are met, the patient should be classified as having FM, regardless of other legitimate medical diagnoses.

Not all patients considered to have FM meet the formal ACR criteria at all times. They can be diagnosed with FM at some times and not at others, according to ACR criteria.

Katz et al argued that FM is a trait, not a state, and a diagnosis is permanent with cooling-off periods and flares. They can have "a little" or no FM and much more at other times.[19] They found fault with the ACR criteria in that they rely too heavily on pain symptoms, the dominant but not the only characteristic of FM. It also is not an objective measure and it could be argued that the 11-point cutoff is truly arbitrary. There is plenty of potential for malingering or false reporting of symptoms. Katz et al proposed a survey that included assessments of demographic features; comorbid illness; disability status; a review of symptoms; the Health Assessment Questionnaire II; the Short Form 36 mood score; and Visual Analog Scale for pain, fatigue, sleep problems, and global severity. They found moderate concordance of ACR and survey criteria (72.3%).[19]

The survey method clearly appears to be more comprehensive than the ACR criteria. It addresses most of the symptoms of FM and correlates significantly with dysfunction. So, should this be the gold standard of FM diagnosis? Perhaps. Is it practical in the modern physical therapy setting? There is no mention of how much time the survey takes and a survey does not take any measures to reduce or eliminate false reporting or malingering. Katz et al mentioned that one advantage of the survey method is that the clinician does not have to touch the patient. Is that a positive thing? Although some pain may be elicited, the ACR exam is not a very painful assessment and, if done properly, may even be a first step in forming a trusting relationship between the patient and practitioner. A tender touch and empathy will signal to the patient that the practitioner understands the pain that FM can cause. While performing the examination, the practitioner is given the opportunity to also assess skin, posture, muscle tone, and even anxiety levels. One thing is for sure: the ACR method takes 2 to 3 min to complete. It is concise and conclusive.

FM is only one of many soft tissue pain syndromes. Accordingly, numerous authors have outlined a classification system to determine the presence of the diagnosis[3,11,15]:

- Local
  - Bursitis: Subacromial, olecranon, trochanteric, prepatellar, anserine
  - Tenosynovitis: Biceps, supraspinatus, infrapatellar, Achilles
  - Enthesopathies: Lateral epicondylitis, medial epicondylitis
- Regional
  - Myofascial pain syndrome: Involving muscles of the trunk and extremities
  - Myofascial pain dysfunction syndrome: Myofascial pain syndrome involving facial muscles
  - Referred pain: Pain referred from visceral and other soft tissue sites

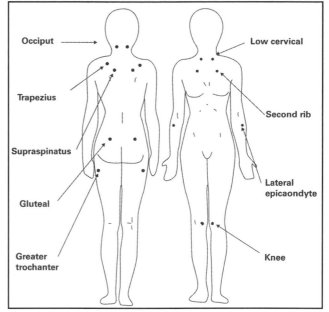

Figure 7-2. ACR FM criteria. (Adapted from Kaltsas G, Tsiveriotis K. Fibromyalgia. In: Chrousos G, ed. *Adrenal Physiology and Diseases*. South Dartmouth: MA: MDText.com; 2013. http://www.endotext.org/adrenal/adrenal33/adrenal33.htm.)

  - Complex regional pain syndrome: Types I and II
- Generalized
  - FM
  - Chronic fatigue syndrome: FM-like when widespread body pain present
  - Osteomalacia: Vitamin D deficiency
  - Hypermobility syndrome: Soft tissue laxity in axial skeleton and joints

Each of these syndromes presents in different degrees and intensities. They each respond differently to medications and exercise. Each one should be managed with the appropriate specific evidence-based protocol. Exercise on land and in water is prescribed for each of these conditions and, for the sake of this text, the protocols described should be considered appropriate and safe. As with any condition, diagnosis, or dysfunction, a comprehensive physical therapy assessment should be performed before any treatment is prescribed. In addition, treatment should be specific to the physical and functional deficits of the patient.

MANAGEMENT OF FIBROMYALGIA

Because there are physical, emotional, chemical, and cognitive components to FM, a multidisciplinary approach appears to be the most effective manner of managing FM.[20-23] Strong evidence supports aerobic exercise and cognitive–behavioral therapy. Moderate evidence supports manual therapy (Figure 7-3), muscle strength training,

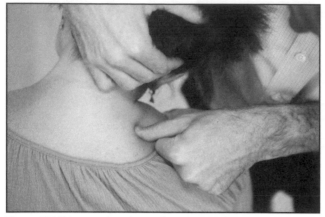

Figure 7-3. Trigger point release of upper trapezius.

acupuncture, and spa therapy (balneotherapy). Limited evidence supports spinal manipulation, movement/body awareness, vitamins, herbs, and dietary modification.[24] Medications and psychosocial interventions combined with exercise seem to produce the most positive health effects. To be successful, any FM program requires that the patient be an active participant in his or her treatment.

The acronym ADEPT Living[25] has been used to help practitioners remember the 6 main categories of intervention:

- Attitude
- Diagnosis
- Education
- Physical activity
- Treatments
- Living

The attitudes of the patient, family members, and practitioners all contribute to the patient's ability to manage FM. On some days, movement and normal daily activities will be intolerable, whereas others are much less painful. This can be frustrating, discouraging, and even confusing to the patient and those around them. Understanding and accepting the often unpredictable natural ebb and flow of FM can minimize some of the stress-related symptoms.

The patient's physicians, therapists, and other health care providers play an ever-present role in a patient's ability to manage his or her FM. If the patient feels stigmatized, he or she will be more reluctant to actively participate in his or her own care. Many health professionals still do not accept FM as a legitimate diagnosis or condition. Empathy will be more therapeutic than baseless recrimination.[17] A supportive and helpful health care team is fundamental to the patient's successful management of FM.

An accurate diagnosis is essential to appropriate treatment of FM. Patients with FM will often describe relief with finally being diagnosed. Without an explanation for the way they feel, the symptoms they are experiencing, and the

life-altering effects, the syndrome is compounded. Some practitioners are unwilling to stamp a patient with the label of FM because they either do not recognize it as a legitimate diagnosis or they do not know how to treat it. This reluctance only hinders a patient's road to recovery until he or she is correctly diagnosed.

Effective education of patients with FM tends to focus on basic knowledge of the syndrome, relaxation training, behavior modification, and pain and stress management. Active management is encouraged. In effective programs, patients are expected to understand the behaviors that improve and exacerbate their symptoms. Cognitive–behavioral therapy has been shown to improve pain scores, pain coping, pain behavior, depression, and physical function.[26–30] Patients should be informed of their treatment options and assured that FM is a manageable condition. If they do follow the treatment protocol, their symptoms will remain under control and they will be able to live a normal and productive life.

Physical activity levels directly impact the effect of FM on anyone afflicted with the condition. Inactivity, more than anything else, tends to aggravate FM in patients and feed into the cycle of decreased perceived physical function. Patients should be encouraged to be more active. In their 2010 study, Fontaine et al[31] followed a specific protocol to meet the guidelines of the US Surgeon General's 1996 Physical Activity Recommendations.[32] The participants in the study were all minimally active prior to enrollment. Initially, they were asked to perform 15 min, above their usual level, of accumulated moderate-intensity lifestyle physical activity (LPA), 5 to 7 days per week, and to increase that amount by 5 min each week. LPA can consist of walking, yard work, using the stairs, exercise, and other physical activity. After getting to 30 min per day, they were free to accumulate more LPA but not required to. The study found that 30 min per day, 5 to 7 days per week, above one's usual activity, of moderate-intensity LPA produced clinically relevant changes in perceived physical function and pain in previously minimally active adults with FM.[31]

On the other end of the activity spectrum, FM patients should also be advised to not overdo their daily activity levels. Excessive lifting or exertion over a prolonged period of time can worsen FM symptoms as well. Pacing of LPA, working for short periods of time followed by an equal amount of rest, can be very effective in avoiding overexertion. This method can be employed to gradually increase LPA to the prescribed 30 min daily. It is not required that the 30 min be done consecutively but that it accumulate throughout the day. Small bouts of activity might be less taxing and easier to initiate and sustain over time.

Along with LPA, patients who are able to exercise experience less negative impact of FM in their lives.[25,33] Moderately intense aerobic exercise can improve physical function and self-efficacy, the belief that one can perform a task or behavior.[34] Walking, pool exercise, jogging, and strength training have all proven to be effective interventions for patients with FM. The exception to this is high-intensity exercise programs. If taken beyond the patient with FM's capacity, he or she will experience increased pain and other symptoms. More important, studies have shown significantly higher drop-out rates in high-intensity programs.[35] Because movement and exercise are key, we need to maintain a framework that encourages participation first. Exercise programs should be tailored to the patient's baseline function, symptom severity, and tolerance of exercise-induced pain.[36] Programs should start at levels just below the participant's capacity and the duration and intensity should gradually increase until the participant is exercising at the low end of moderate intensity for 20 to 30 min.[37]

Patients with FM tend to be less active than the rest of the population. Many patients with FM are fearful of moving and being active, because too much activity tends to increase their symptoms. Conversely, symptoms are worsened further by a lack of movement, activity, and exercise. LPA and exercise should be promoted by taking small steps. Focus should initially be on what the patient is comfortable participating in and progression should continue slowly into additional tolerable LPA and exercises. Overexertion should continue to be avoided. In a qualitative study, most women living with FM claimed that they tried to be careful about exceeding their limits with respect to physical activity because of subsequently "paying for it," describing a worsening of FM symptoms postexercise.[38] Nonetheless, the value of exercise should be emphasized and is a part of every successful FM management protocol.

Pharmacological treatment of FM is an essential element in most programs. There are several effective pharmacological interventions for patients with FM. Because this is a text focused on aquatic physical therapy, this chapter will not delve deeply into pharmacological agents except to mention the effective classes of medications. Certain analgesics, other than nonsteroidal anti-inflammatory drugs, can be effective. Precursors, biogenic amine reuptake inhibitors, serotonin receptor blockades, N-methyl-D-aspartate receptor blockades, anticonvulsants, and sedatives have all shown some effectiveness in the treatment of FM.[13] It also should be noted that there is no specific surgery for the treatment of FM.

AQUATIC THERAPY FOR PATIENTS WITH FIBROMYALGIA

The physical therapist has many tools to guide patients in their management of FM. None has proven to be more effective than the therapy pool.[39] The properties of water create a comfortable environment for patients with severe chronic pain to relax, move, and exercise with significantly reduced symptoms. During that time, they are able to comfortably exercise more vigorously than on dry land. Aquatic therapy is one of the most effective means of initiating an exercise program and helping patients with FM to be compliant over the long term. The warmth of a heated pool helps lubricate joints and loosens muscles. Patients find it easy to move freely and tolerate longer bursts of exercise with minimal residual soreness or increases in pain. Moreover, patients typically report that the relief from being in a heated pool and performing aquatic exercise tends to last for hours.

Munguia-Izquierdo and Legaz-Arrese found that an exercise therapy program with moderate intensity performed 3 times a week for 16 weeks in a chest-high pool of warm water (32°C) has no apparent negative effects and improves pain, sleep quality, and physical and cognitive function, resulting in adherence to exercise in previously unfit women with heightened and long FM symptomatology.[40] This shows that aquatic therapy achieves the major objectives of an FM exercise program: increased function, relief of the predominant symptoms, and patient adherence to a program.

Patients who are otherwise fearful of exercise can participate in aquatic therapy without the usual postexercise symptoms. They can perform aerobic and resistance exercises with decreased potential to injure themselves. Aquatic therapy has been found to be a safe and beneficial mode of exercise that can be performed as part of a well-rounded exercise program.[41] The margin of therapeutic safety is wider than that of almost any other treatment milieu.[42]

The buoyancy of water significantly reduces the effective body weight on the patient. Shoulder-height water reduces the effect of gravity on the patient's body by 80%, effectively making a 200-lb person feel as if he or she weighs approximately 40 lbs. This lighter feeling increases freedom of movement, decreases pain, and psychologically helps the patient by relieving her of the constant pain that she normally experiences. Buoyancy is of great therapeutic value to someone with a chronic pain syndrome that is exacerbated by weight bearing.

The viscous properties of water create a unique exercise environment. Slow movement is facilitated by the combination of buoyancy and minimal viscosity. As the speed of movement increases, resistance increases as a log function of velocity. Increased velocity of movement requires greater force, producing a gentle, even resistance that works as a strengthener without painful side effects. Viscous resistance increases as more force is exerted, but that resistance drops to 0 almost instantaneously when a person stops movement.[42] This allows enhanced control of strengthening activities within the envelope of patient comfort.[43] Consider also that the viscosity of water means that there is no risk of dropping a weight on one's foot, overexertion is improbable, and there is minimal risk of gravity forcing a joint into an angle beyond the normal range of motion. These positive attributes all contribute

Figure 7-4. Aquatic treadmill ambulation.

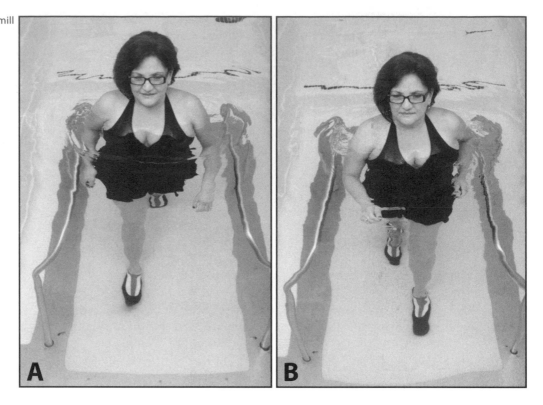

to the safe environment of an aquatic exercise program, helping the patient with FM overcome the roadblocks that lead to the avoidance of exercise, making her more likely to participate.

Patients with FM are hypersensitive to touch, pressure, and temperature. A warm pool of water reacts positively to each of these sensations. Water feels soothing on the skin; hydrostatic pressure exerts an even, gentle force to the entire body; and the warmth of a 33.5°C to 35.5°C therapeutic pool soothes aching joints and muscles. The thermal conductive property, combined with the high specific heat of water, makes the use of water in rehabilitation very versatile because water retains heat or cold while delivering it easily to the immersed body.[42]

This text will elaborate on physical therapy in a warm pool (33.5°C to 35.5°C) with a treadmill (Figure 7-4) built into the floor of the pool. Because aerobic exercise is considered the most effective physical therapy intervention for FM, an aquatic treadmill is an ideal tool to achieve aerobic level output in a safe, minimal-impact environment. Rife et al found water treadmill running to be an effective alternative to land treadmill running, comparable to land-based running while minimizing impact forces.[39] Buoyancy reduces the metabolic demands of exercising in water, increasing the patient's hang time while running and decreasing physical effort and heart rate. In order to obtain an equivalent cardiorespiratory overload of land treadmill running, individuals should select a water treadmill running speed that elicits a heart rate of approximately 7 bpm less than their typical land treadmill running heart rate.

Rife et al also found that due to added drag, water shoes increase the metabolic demand on any given water treadmill speed.[44]

Tomas-Carus et al studied the effects of a long-term (8 months) aquatic therapy program on women with FM. They showed that these patients exhibited improvements in physical and mental health at a magnitude similar to those patients in shorter programs.[45] This program employed low-intensity exercise and does not detail any exercise progressions. Although no significant improvements were made for most subjects once a threshold was met, patients continued to experience relief and improvement in their pain and functional levels. From this we can conclude that patients with FM can tolerate an aquatics program over the long term and they are willing to continue participation.

In our current third-party payer environment, long-term aquatic therapy treatment may not be feasible. In reality, this intervention is more suited to a wellness model, which many physical therapy practices are moving toward, particularly for patients with chronic conditions who require continued care. In fact, this may be an ideal scenario for patient and provider, one that should be considered in all aquatic centers with a population of patients with FM.

Different standards have been used in studies of aquatic exercise for FM. Several met the minimum standards of the American College of Sports Medicine.[22,40,46] Another study made sure that the patients performed all exercises with awareness and were taught how to modify the exercises to match their own threshold of pain and fatigue. Only when patients were able to perform the movements

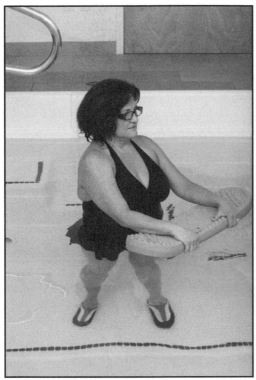

Figure 7-5. Trunk rotation left.

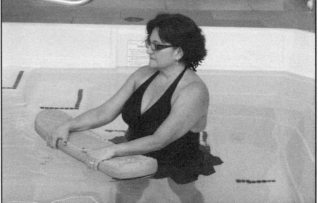

Figure 7-6. Trunk rotation right.

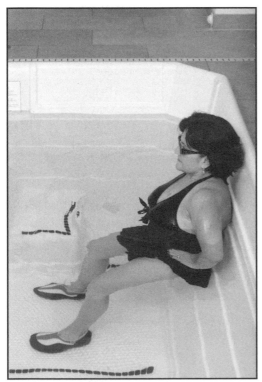

Figure 7-7. Wall squat.

in a harmonious flow were they encouraged to increase the pace and the load of exercises to attain cardiovascular and strength training.[47] In another study, exercise was not intended as training. The intensity and repetitions were self-selected, and participants never reached their pain or fatigue threshold. The success of this program suggests that though training volume is an important focus for improving cardiorespiratory fitness, this may not be so for the effective management of FM symptoms.[48]

Most documented programs consist of approximately 1 hour of exercise broken down into a warm-up, mobility and stretching, strengthening, core and balance exercises, functional activities, higher intensity aerobic training, and cool down (Figures 7-5 to 7-11). This program is similar to a general conditioning program or a program tailored to patients with severe arthritis. Practitioners and patients should be aware that FM patients often do not experience severe symptoms during activity, particularly once integrated into a program and exercising regularly. They may develop a false sense of security and attempt to push themselves far beyond what they have done in the past. This can lead to days of increased pain and hesitancy to progress their program any time in the near future. Gradual progression is a key to successful exercise. The aquatic environment is a bit more forgiving than dry-land exercise, but it is very important that the patient and physical therapist know the progression tolerance so that the patient can advance safely.

CONCLUSION

FM is a complicated syndrome that affects the entire life of a patient afflicted with it. With proper multidisciplinary care and active patient involvement, the symptoms can be managed and the patient can maintain control of her life. An active lifestyle, including daily exercise, is an integral part of FM management. Aquatic therapy is an effective component of any FM program.

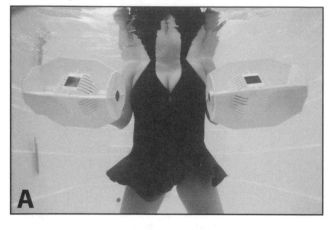

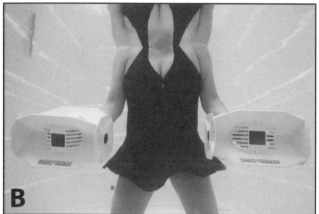

Figure 7-8. Bicep curls with Hydro-Bells (Hydro-Tone Fitness Systems, Inc, Yorba Linda, CA).

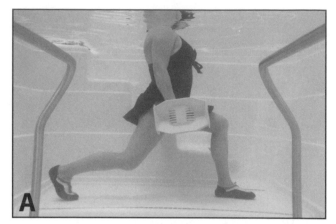

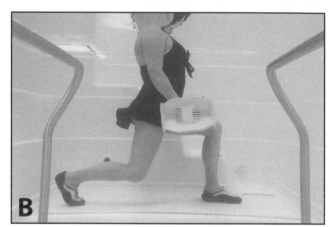

Figure 7-9. Lunges with Hydro-Bells.

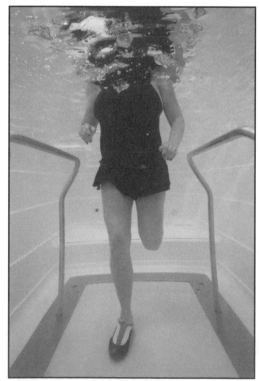

Figure 7-10. Jogging on treadmill.

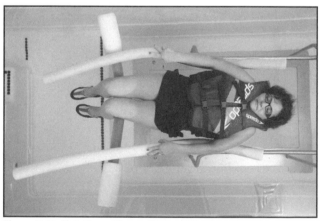

Figure 7-11. Flotation with noodles and vest.

References

1. Schmidt-Wilcke T, Luerding R, Weigand T, et al. Striatal grey matter increase in patients suffering from fibromyalgia—a voxel-based morphometry study. *Pain.* 2007;132(suppl):109–116.
2. Buskila D. Developments in the scientific and clinical understanding of fibromyalgia. *Arthritis Res Ther.* 2009;11:242–252.
3. Wolfe F, Smythe HA, Yunus MB, et al. The American College of Rheumatology 1990 criteria for the classification of fibromyalgia: report of the Multicenter Criteria Committee. *Arthritis Rheum.* 1990;33:160–172.

4. Henriksson C, Gundmark I, Bengtsson A, Ek AC. Living with fibromyalgia. Consequences of everyday life. *Clin J Pain.* 1992;8:138–144.

5. Waylonis GW, Ronan PG, Gordon C. Fibromyalgia in occupational environments. *Am J Phys Med Rehabil.* 1994;73:112–115.

6. Mengshoel AM, Forre O, Komnaes HB. Muscle strength and aerobic capacity in primary fibromyalgia. *Clin Exp Rheumatol.* 1990;8:475–479.

7. Nordenskiöld UM, Grimby G. Grip force in patients with rheumatoid arthritis, fibromyalgia and in healthy subjects. A study with a Grippit instrument. *Scand J Rheumatol.* 1993;22:14–19.

8. Mannerkorpi K, Burckhardt CS, Bjelle A. Physical performance characteristics of women with fibromyalgia. *Arthritis Care Res.* 1994;7:123–129.

9. Jones KD, Burckhardt CS, Clark SR, Bennett RM, Potempa KM. A randomized controlled trial of muscle strengthening versus flexibility training in fibromyalgia. *J Rheumatol.* 2002;29:1041-1048.

10. Inanici F, Yunus MB. History of fibromyalgia: past to present. *Curr Pain Headache Rep.* 2004;8:369–378.

11. Wolf F, Ross K, Anderson J, Russell IJ, Hebert L. The prevalence and characteristics of fibromyalgia in the general population. *Arthritis Rheum.* 1995;38:19–28.

12. Akers D, Eyer S. *Living With Fibromyalgia: A Journey of Hope and Understanding* [DVD]. San Francisco, CA: Trillusion Media; 2006.

13. Bradley LA, Alarcon GS, Sotolongo A, et al. Cerebrospinal fluid (CSF) levels of substance P (SP) are abnormal in patients with fibromyalgia (FM) regardless of traumatic or insidious pain onset. *Arthritis Rheum.* 1998;41(suppl):S256.

14. Russell IJ. Elevated cerebrospinal fluid levels of substance P in patients with the fibromyalgia syndrome. *Arthritis Rheum.* 1994;37:1593–1601.

15. Pellegrino M. *Fibromyalgia: Up Close and Personal.* Columbus, OH: Anadem Publishing; 2005.

16. Chakrabarty S, Zoorob R. Fibromyalgia. *Am Fam Physician.* 2007;76:247–254.

17. Wolfe F. Diagnosis of fibromyalgia: the new criteria. *J Musculoskelet Med.* 1990;7:53–69.

18. Wolfe F. Pain extent and diagnosis: development and validation of the regional pain scale in 12,799 patients with rheumatic disease. *J Rheumatol.* 2003;30:369–378.

19. Katz RS, Wolfe F, Michaud K. Fibromyalgia diagnosis: a comparison of clinical, survey, and American College of Rheumatology criteria. *Arthitis Rheum.* 2006;54:169–176.

20. Lemstra M, Olszynski WP. The effectiveness of multidisciplinary rehabilitation in the treatment of fibromyalgia. *Clin J Pain.* 2005;21(2):166–174.

21. Cedraschi C, Desmeules J, Rapiti E, et al. Fibromyalgia: a randomized, controlled trial of a treatment programme based on self management. *Ann Rheum Dis.* 2004;63:2906.

22. Busch AJ, Schachter CL, Overend TJ, Peloso PM, Barbare KAR. Exercise for fibromyalgia: a systematic review. *J Rheumatol.* 2008;35:1130–1144.

23. Burckhardt CS, Mannerkorpi K, Hedenberg L, Bjelle A. A randomized, controlled clinical trial of education and physical training for women with fibromyalgia. *J Rheumatol.* 1994;21:714–720.

24. Schneider M, Vernon H, Ko G, Lawson G, Perera J. Chiropractic management of fibromyalgia syndrome: a systematic review of the literature. *J Manipulative Physiol Ther.* 2009;32(1):25–40.

25. Russell IJ, Raphael KG. Fibromyalgia syndrome: approach to management. *CNS Spectr.* 2008;13(suppl 5):6–11.

26. Burckhardt CS. Nonpharmalogic management strategies in fibromyalgia. *Rheum Dis Clin North Am.* 2002;28:291–304.

27. Vlaeyen JW, Teeken-Gruben NJ, Goosens ME. Cognitive-educational treatment of fibromyalgia: a randomized clinical trial. *J Rheumatol.* 1996;25:77–86.

28. Karjalainen K, Malmivaara A, van Tulder M, et al. Multidisciplinary rehabilitation for fibromyalgia and musculoskeletal pain in working age adults. *The Cochrane Libr.* 2001;2:1–33.

29. Rossy LA, Buckelew SP, Dorr N, et al. A meta-analysis of fibromyalgia treatment interventions. *Ann Behav Med.* 1999;21:180–191.

30. Sim J, Adams N. Systematic review of randomized controlled trials of nonpharmalogical interventions for fibromyalgia. *Clin J Pain.* 2002;18:324–336.

31. Fontaine KR, Conn L, Clauw DJ. Effects of lifestyle physical activity on perceived symptoms and physical function in adults with fibromyalgia: results of a randomized trial. *Arthritis Res Ther.* 2010;12(2):R55.

32. United States Department of Health and Human Services, Physical Activity and Health. A report to the Surgeon General. Atlanta, GA: US Department of Health and Human Services, Centers for Disease Control and Prevention, National Center for Chronic Disease Prevention and Health Promotion; 1996.

33. Gowans SE, deHueck A. Pool exercise for individuals with fibromyalgia. *Curr Opin Rheumatol.* 2007;19:168–173.

34. Lorig K, Chastain RL, Ung E, et al. Development and valuation of a scale to measure perceived self-efficacy in people with arthritis. *Arthritis Rheum.* 1989;32:37–44.

35. Jones KD, Adams D, Winters-Stone K, Burckhardt CS. A comprehensive review of 46 exercise treatment studies in fibromyalgia (1988–2005). *Health Qual Life Outcomes.* 2006;4:67–72.

36. Mannerkorpi K. Exercise in fibromyalgia. *Curr Opin Rheumatol.* 2005;17:190–194.

37. Gowans SE, deHueck A. Exercise for fibromyalgia: benefits and practical advice. *J Musculoskelet Med.* 2006;23:614–622.

38. Busch AJ, Thille P, Barber KAR, Schachter CL, Bidonde J, Collacott BK. Best practice: e-model—prescribing physical activity and exercise for individuals with fibromyalgia. *Physiother Theory Pract.* 2008;24(3):151–166.

39. Evcik D, Yigit I, Pusak I, Kavuncu V. Effectiveness of aquatic therapy in the treatment of fibromyalgia syndrome: a randomized controlled open study. *Rheumatol Int.* 2008;28:885–890.

40. Munguia-Izquierdo D, Legaz-Arrese A. Assessment of the effects of aquatic therapy in global symptomatology in patients with fibromyalgia syndrome: a randomized controlled trial. *Arch Phys Med Rehabil.* 2008;89:2250–2257.

41. Takeshima N, Rogers ME, Watanabe E, et al. Water-based exercise improves health-related aspects of fitness in older women. *Appl Sci.* 2002;34:544–551.

42. Becker BE. Aquatic therapy: scientific foundations and clinical rehabilitation applications. *PM R.* 2009;1:859–872.

43. Poyhonen T, Keskinen KL, Hautala A, Malkia E. Determination of hydrodynamic drag forces and drag coefficients on human leg/foot model during knee extension. *Clin Biomech.* 2000;15:256–260.

44. Rife RK, Myrer JW, Vehrs P, Feland JB, Hunter I, Fellingham GW. Water treadmill parameters needed to obtain land treadmill intensities in runners. *Med Sci Sports Exerc.* 2009;42:733–738.

45. Tomas-Carus P, Gusi N, Hakkinen A, Hakkinen K, Leal A, Ortega-Alonso A. Eight months of physical training in warm water improves physical and mental health in women with fibromyalgia: a randomized controlled trial. *J Rehabil Med.* 2008;40:248–252.

46. American College of Sports Medicine. *ACSM's Guidelines for Exercise Testing and Prescription.* 7th ed. Philadelphia: Lippincott, Williams & Wilkins; 2006.

47. Mannerkorpi K, Ahlmen M, Ekdahl C. Six and 24-month follow-up of pool exercise therapy and education for patients with fibromyalgia. *Scand J Rheumatol.* 2002;31:306–310.

48. Mannerkorpi K, Nyberg B, Ahlmen M, Ekdahl C. Pool exercise combined with an education program for patients with fibromyalgia syndrome: a prospective, randomized study. *J Rheumatol.* 2000;27:2473–2481.

Section III

Conditioning and Training

8

Strength Training and Conditioning

Murphy Grant, MS, ATC, NASM-PES, CES

The world of sports performance, personal training, athletic conditioning, and performance enhancement is constantly changing. This thought process along with an aquatic medium will keep sport and fitness enthusiasts on the cutting edge of injury prevention, fitness, and performance enhancement. When designing and implementing strength training exercises in any workout, there needs be a development of all fitness and health components, such as functional strength, flexibility, nutritional efficiency, and metabolic efficiency, because this will aid in achieving peak performance. Strength training results in improvements in strength, speed, power, agility, endurance, neuromuscular control, and flexibility. One of the basic aspects of most exercise prescriptions in training programs is related to improving the body's ability to gain energy.[1]

The purpose of this chapter is to present a rationale for aquatic-based strength training and explain why it can have significant strength benefits, even with elite athletes. However, aquatic strength and power training should not be a replacement for land-based strength training but a supplement, an adjunct to land-based therapy to help develop strength and power in athletes.

The health-related benefits of strength training are profound, such as potential improvement in cardiovascular efficiency, decreased body fat, increased tensile muscle strength, increased bone density, and an improved psychological profile.[2] The benefits of an aquatic medium will help develop a solid strength base in which power (speed–strength) can be enhanced. A solid strength base also protects the body against future injuries.

Although there is a need for stronger, more powerful athletes, it is important to emphasize that there are different types of strength. Each athlete has different strength needs based upon sport position and role on the team (for team sports). Additionally, there are certain training prerequisites necessary to safely build explosive strength and power. It is imperative to have appropriate mobility and stabilizer strength prior to developing prime-mover strength and endurance, which in turn must be developed prior to adding power, explosiveness, speed, and agility.[3]

Focusing on explosive strength and power prior to developing mobility, stability, endurance, and speed would potentially be deleterious to athletic performance.

Athletes who take this approach often have poor balance and stability, may sustain an injury, and ultimately may perform poorly in competition due to a lack of functional strength and power. Aquatic strength training, if used as a supplement to land-based resistance training, can help address limitations in the mobility, stability, and endurance, thus helping build maximal strength and power. The unique properties of water allow for what may be termed constant functional resistance. Every movement made in the water is resisted, and as the velocity of the movement increases, the resistance increases exponentially.

Due to the exponential relationship between velocity of movement in the water and amount of resistance (created from drag) received, it becomes clear how aquatic strength training can be a highly effective tool in developing all types of strength, including stabilizer, maximal, power, and functional. The faster a segment moves in water, the more resistance there is to overcome. This is due to the fact that drag is velocity dependent or, more precisely, velocity squared. This implies that if you double the velocity you

Wilk KE, Joyner DM. *The Use of Aquatics in Orthopedic and Sports Medicine Rehabilitation and Physical Conditioning* (pp 93-102).
© 2014 SLACK Incorporated.

move in water, the resistive drag force increases by a factor of 4.

The concept of strength training has existed since the days of Hippocrates; consequently, people have developed different ways to enhance athletes' abilities to perform work. Strength is the ability to perform work. One thing that performance enhancement and rehabilitation professionals agree on is that we are constantly seeking ways to help athletes produce the most amount of work with the least amount of effort as quickly as possible.

This can be further illustrated by considering the equations for work (W = F [force] × D [distance]) and power (P = W/t [time]). The ability to perform work and power is enhanced by manipulating the variables in these equations. By increasing F or D or decreasing t we can increase W and P. As strength increases, power potentially increases.

When manipulating the F, D, or t variables to get increased W or P, athletes need to train in a manner that maximizes strength and power. To maximize strength gains, it is important to understand and apply the basic principles of strength training, which include progressive overload, specificity, reversibility, fitness, rest intervals, and recovery.

The basic premise of progressive overload is to progressively increase the load on the musculoskeletal system. Once muscles, tendons, ligaments, and bones adapt to a given stimuli, additional loads must be placed on these structures for further adaptation to occur. This is often done by small increases in load and keeping the repetitions the same or by larger increases in load and at the same time decreasing the number of repetitions performed. The overload principle can be manipulated by varying several factors such as exercise intensity, duration, volume, frequency, rest intervals, mode, and periodization.

Training intensity is commonly synonymous with the resistance being overcome. The higher the resistance, the higher the training intensity. Training studies have shown that strength is maximized by employing heavy resistance between a 3 repitition maximum (RM; heaviest weight performed for 3 consecutive repetitions) and 8 RM.[3] Therefore, it is common for strength training programs to employ multiple sets between 3 and 8 repetitions. In the water, resistance can be increased by using larger implements (eg, water dumbbells or paddles) with greater surface area and by increasing movement velocity. Moderate intensities between 8 and 12 RM intensities develop moderate strength gains, whereas performing beyond 12 repetitions is considered low-intensity training, which changes the emphasis from muscular strength to muscular endurance.

Training intensity can also be quantified and expressed as the power output generated while performing an exercise. Power is defined as work per unit time. Since Work = (Force)(Distance), and Speed = Distance/Time, Power can be expressed as the product of force and speed (otherwise termed strength–speed) as follows: Power = (Work/Time) = [(Force)(Distance)/Time] = (Force)(Speed). To maximize power, it is important to train in a way that maximizes the rate of force development (RFD), which is the speed at which force can be produced. The shorter the time interval in which force can be produced, the faster the RFD and the greater the amount of power developed. RFD can be enhanced by using a variety of different training systems.[3] Examples of training systems include resistance training with high movement speeds and light loads, heavy loads and slow movement speeds, and static contractions with the intention of a high RFD. It appears that an increase in RFD is most efficiently found through different combinations of training.[3]

There are different modes of training that can be used to maximize strength and power. One mode of training that has been linked to successfully increasing RFD, strength, and power is the use of bands and chains. The basic idea here is that bands and chains allow us to manipulate the F variable in the W = F × D equation to increase work and power. As you move the band or chain further through the range of motion, resistance increases and, therefore, more force is required. The increasing resistance allows the lifter to accelerate through the entire range of motion without having to decelerate or coast to the finish. It is less about the speed at which the movement is produced and more about intent or attempt to move the resistance as fast as possible through the entire range of motion. Bands and chains are just a way of stimulating the muscle in a different way and manipulating the force–velocity curve.

One mode of training that has been linked to successful enhancement of lower and upper body power production and vertical jump performance is plyometric training.[3,4] It has been demonstrated that aquatic-based plyometric training can increase vertical jump performance in volleyball players.[4] In plyometric training, movements should be explosive, with the athlete being instructed to move as fast as possible through the water.

One common denominator between plyometric training and training with bands or chains is that they each result in muscles being trained under greater tensions for longer periods through the strength curve than can be achieved through conventional resistance training. In an aquatic median, this potentially may be related to the fundamental fact that the drag properties of water affect muscles at different points along the force–velocity curve and, therefore, different training adaptations may occur. As introduced earlier, this manipulation of the force–velocity curve is the basis behind the success of training with bands and chains.

One of the drawbacks to land-based power training (plyometrics, bands/chains, etc) is the complaint of reported muscle/joint soreness experienced after sessions. In a study by Robinson et al,[5] the authors compared the effects of land versus aquatic plyometrics on power, torque, velocity, and muscle soreness. The results suggested that aquatic plyometic training can provide the same performance enhancement benefits as land-based programs but with significantly less muscle soreness. These findings suggest that athletes can develop the same levels of power with less muscle soreness, minimizing noncontact injury risk.

The highest power outputs recorded in sport activities occur in lifting maximum or near maximum loads during the snatch and clean and jerk exercises during weight lifting competition.[6] These types of exercises are performed explosively, generating high force and power outputs. Explosive training with moderate to heavy loads produces maximum fast twitch fiber recruitment, which is important because the peak power output of fast twitch fibers is about 4 times as great as in slow twitch fibers.[7] Explosive power training, especially combined with strength training, also increases motor unit synchronization and the RFD.[8]

Training volume for any given exercise is determined by multiplying the total number of sets, repetitions, and resistance.[9] Typically, volume increases as intensity decreases, and volume decreases as intensity increases. Because a force is being applied to an implement as it moves through a given distance, training volume is also a measure of the total mechanical work performed during an exercise or training session.

Rest interval refers to the total rest time between repetitions, sets, and exercises for a given muscle group being worked. When training a specific muscle group, a 2- to 3-min rest interval between sets is common in strength training, often increasing with increasing intensities (eg, 4- to 5-min rest interval for >90% 1 RM training intensities) and decreasing with decreasing intensities (eg, 1- to 2-min rest interval for 70% to 80% 1 RM training intensities and 30- to 60-sec rest interval for 40% to 60% 1 RM training intensity). The increase in rest intervals with higher intensity training compared to lower intensity training is necessary in part due to the greater number of motor units recruited and a larger accumulation of lactate and to allow complete recovery when training with near maximal loads. In addition, multi-muscle, multi-joint exercises (eg, squats, power cleans, bench presses), which require a large energy expenditure, require longer rest times than single-muscle, single-joint exercises (eg, leg extensions, leg curls, arm curls), which have a much lower energy expenditure.

Rest intervals are also needed between exercise sessions in order to allow time for muscle and connective tissue to repair and regenerate from training. Compared to low-intensity training, high-intensity training causes more muscle and connective tissue damage and requires greater time to repair and regenerate.[10] Typically, 48 to 72 hours is needed between training sessions for muscle and connective tissue muscle to adequately recover.[10] Adequate rest and protein intake are 2 of the most common factors for muscle regeneration. Research has shown that a protein intake of 1.5 to 2 g/kg body mass is most effective in muscle regeneration after high-intensity resistance training.[11]

Larger muscles groups, such as the back and hip extensors, often require a longer rest period between training sessions compared to smaller muscle groups, especially those that move through a smaller range of motion (eg, rectus abdominis, which may be trained daily with varying intensities and volume). A commonly employed rest interval protocol for any given muscle group is training on alternating days.

Training duration refers to the total quantity of time during resistance exercise and will vary depending on the type of strength training that is being performed. As the number of exercises, repetitions, sets, and rest intervals increase within a session, training duration will also increase. A typical strength training session lasts between 20 and 60 min. Training duration also refers to the number of weeks or months that a given strength training program is adhered to. A strength training program will typically last 6 to 12 weeks before intensity, duration, frequency, or mode is modified.

Training frequency refers to how often an athlete engages in a strength training program. It is often expressed as total number of training sessions per week. Although strength training once per week can build or maintain strength,[12] it has been demonstrated that strength gains are maximized when training occurs during 2 to 3 sessions per week.[12] Despite the evidence that performing multiple strength training sessions per week is superior in producing strength gains compared to performing a single strength training session each week, it should be emphasized that single weekly sessions are still efficacious. The single weekly strength training session may be preferred by individuals who have time constraints and whose goals are not to maximize strength gains. It should be emphasized that the intensity of training is more important than duration or frequency of training in maintaining strength gains.[13]

For high-level athletes and deconditioned individuals, it is not uncommon to split a larger training session involving several muscle groups into multiple shorter training sessions throughout the week involving only 1 or 2 muscle groups. This is referred to as split-routine training. A large training session may also be split into multiple shorter training sessions throughout the day. An advantage of splitting a larger training session into multiple shorter sessions is to decrease the physiological and psychological fatigue that accompanies long sessions. A split routine allows an athlete to devote full effort and intensity for each muscle group. The same principles are true for a deconditioned individual training the entire body by performing 3 sets of 8 exercises 3 times per week. This individual may elect to perform 4 upper body exercises in the morning and the remaining 4 lower body exercises in the evening or perform 4 upper body exercises one day and the remaining 4 lower body exercises the following day.

When muscles and connective tissues are given the same stimuli for a prolonged period of time, the strength gains exhibited in these tissues begins to diminish. To continue to stimulate muscles and connective tissues, training intensities, volumes, and exercises must periodically be changed.[14]

This is also important in preventing psychological staleness due to performing the same program for a prolonged period of time. Periodization is a system of training that varies training intensities and volumes throughout a year-long training cycle, referred to as a macrocycle.[14] Periodized training has been shown to produce superior strength and power gains compared to single-set or multi-set training with a constant repetition scheme,[10] even when the training sets and repetitions employed have not been to failure.[15] In addition, periodization training has been shown to increase physical performance abilities in athletes.[15]

A typical macrocycle is broken down into 3 to 4 mesocycles (each 3 to 4 months in duration), and each mesocycle can in turn be broken down into 3 to 4 microcycles (each 3 to 4 weeks in duration). A common periodization pattern for the strength athlete involves beginning a training microcycle with higher volume and lower intensities and progressively increasing intensity and decreasing volume.[14] For example, consider a 4-month mesocycle composed of 4 microcycles of 4 weeks each. The initial 4-week microcycle could involve a higher training volume of 4 sets of 12 repetitions and a lower training intensity of 70% of 1 RM.

This higher volume–lower intensity training microcycle, referred to as the preparatory phase,[14] will gradually allow the muscles and connective tissue to adapt to new stress. In addition, the first microcycle allows the athlete to adapt to performing new exercises that have not recently been performed, with an emphasis on proper lifting form and technique. The strength gains during this initial microcycle will primarily be due to neural factors. The second 4-week microcycle, referred to as the hypertrophy phase,[14] could involve training at 80% 1 RM intensity and decreasing the training volume to 4 sets of 8 repetitions.

The emphasis of this cycle is muscle hypertrophy, which research has shown to be effective when training occurs between approximately 8 to 10 RM (75% to 80% 1 RM).[14] As muscles increase in size, their potential for strength also increases, because the force that a muscle can generate is directly proportional to that muscle's physiological cross-sectional area. The third 4-week microcycle, referred to as the strength phase,[14] could involve training at an 85% to 90% 1 RM intensity and decreasing the training volume to 4 sets of 4 to 6 repetitions.

The emphasis of this cycle is on muscle strength. Upper and lower extremity high-intensity weight training studies have demonstrated significant increases in muscle strength when training between 2 and 12 RM.[13] However, many strength coaches believe that strength is maximized using multiple sets per session, multiple sessions per week, and an intensity between 2 and 6 RM (approximately 85% to 95% 1 RM).

This approach is supported by data from several strength training studies.[14,15] The final 4-week microcycle, referred to as the power phase,[14] could involve training at a 90% to 95% 1 RM intensity and decreasing the training volume to

3 to 5 sets of 2 to 3 repetitions. The emphasis of this cycle is muscle power, which research has shown is maximized in select explosive exercises (ie, clean and jerk, power cleans, snatch) while employing maximal or near maximal loads.[6]

Traditionally speaking, linear periodization is the parent model from which all other models have evolved. This model is termed *linear* due to the calculated gradual increase in intensity over time.[3] An alternative model to linear periodization is undulating or nonlinear. This includes significant changes with each training session in load and volume. An undulating model may be more effective in improving strength than the linear model.[3] The constant changes in load/volume in the undulating model appear to help avoid the neural fatigue often seen with linear models.

Other models of periodization include concurrent and conjugate.[16] Undulating, concurrent, and conjugate models seem to be most appropriately applicable when working with performance athletes.[16] Concurrent periodization is simply training multiple qualities simultaneously. Conjugate is doing the same while additionally linking each training block in an effort to enhance the following one. Aquatic-based strength training falls into these models of training nicely because it provides a unique mode to train multiple qualities of fitness (strength, power, speed, etc) simultaneously while varying load and volume.

Muscles and connective tissue adapt specifically to the demands placed on them. This is known as the specific adaption to imposed demands (SAID) principle. For example, for muscles to hypertrophy, they have to be trained by employing an optimal intensity for that specific adaptation, which, as previously mentioned, is approximately 70% to 80% 1 RM. Similarly, for muscles to maximally adapt to becoming stronger, a higher intensity should be employed (approximately 80% to 95% 1 RM), and for bones to increase in density and become stronger, weight-bearing exercises should be used.

In addition to applying the SAID principle to muscle and connective tissues, the SAID principle applies to exercise selections for sport-specific movements. An example of this is the squat movement, which is specific to jumping in basketball. The squat is also sport specific for American football because it develops the largest and most powerful muscles of the body (ie, gluteals, quadriceps, hamstrings, and erector spinae), which are important in both sprinting and jumping. In addition, an incline bench press follows a path that is more sport specific to the shot put compared to the flat bench press. Moreover, though the power clean is a movement that is sport specific to several positions in American football, it is not a sport-specific movement for overhand throwing and hitting in baseball and could potentially have deleterious effects.

Strength gains are transient and reversible with disuse, with further losses in strength due to disuse occurring at a greater rate than gains in strength due to training.[17]

Table 8-1.

Core Stabilization Concept

Example #1	Example #2
If the extremity muscles are strong and the core is weak, there will not be enough force created to have efficient movements.	A weak core is a fundamental problem due to inefficient movement that leads to injury pattern.

However, as previously outlined, strength gains can be maintained with as little as one strength training session per week as long as high-intensity training is employed.[13]

Unfit individuals achieve strength gains at a faster rate than trained individuals but also lose strength due to disuse at a faster rate than trained individuals.[17] The initial strength gains experienced by unfit individuals are largely due to neural factors such as increased neuromuscular coordination between muscles and decreased sensitivity in the golgi tendon organs.[8,18]

Proper application of the aforementioned principles of strength training results in specific strength training adaptations. High-volume training can result in a decrease in body fat, improved lean muscle mass, increased metabolic efficiency, and increased cross-sectional area of muscle cells. High-intensity training can result in increased neuromuscular coordination and increased motor unit recruitment. All strength training programs should be progressive and systematic because this will prevent overtraining and injury.[2]

Strength training is an essential component of all exercise programs. Because all muscles function eccentrically, isometrically, and concentrically in all 3 planes of motion, strength training programs should utilize a multidimensional/multiplanar approach using the entire muscle contraction and velocity contraction.[3] There are several types of strength that will need to be considered when designing aquatic strength training programs: limit, endurance, maximal, speed, reactive, stabilization, core, and functional (Table 8-1).

Functional strength training raises some controversy: should it be done standing and should it be multi-joint? Function varies from joint to joint; exercises that promote function of a joint requiring stabilizing strength are different from those exercises that promote function of a joint that strives for mobility. When designing strength training programs, it is important to understand how athletes move and what movements are important in their sport. Training should be a vehicle to improve performance and not just strength. With all of the different types of strength, the most important factor is to combine all of these to minimize injury risk and maximize athletic performance.

Table 8-2.

Core Musculature

Local Musculature	• Transverse abdominus
	• Internal oblique
	• Multifidus
	• Lumbar transversospinalis
Global Musculature	• Rectus abdominus
	• External oblique
	• Erector spinae
	• Quadratus lumborum
	• Adductor complex
	• Quadriceps
	• Hamstring
	• Gluteus maximus

There are many different types of systems presently used in strength and conditioning.[3,19] These systems include single-set, circuit training, multiple-set, peripheral heart action, pyramids, supersets and split routines (Table 8-2).

- Single-set (one of the oldest training methods): When one performs one set of each exercise, usually 8 to 12 repetitions.

- Circuit: Performing a series of exercises in which one performs 10 to 15 repetitions one after another with very little rest. This is a great training system for those who have very little time to train and want to alter their body composition.

- Multiple-set: Training that typically consists of performing 2 to 5 sets; warm-up sets of increasing resistance, with additional sets consist of same resistance.

- Peripheral heart action: A variation of circuit training consisting of 4 to 6 exercises for different body parts/regions, with each exercise made up of 8 to 12 repetitions. This training system is great for incorporating multidimensional movement.

- Pyramid: A training program in which an individual performs a light resistance and works to a heavier resistance with each set typically made up of 4 to 6 sets and 10 to 12 repetitions. This system can also be performed in the opposite direction, working from heavier resistance to lower resistance.

- Superset: A great training technique for hypertrophy, consisting of sets of 8 to 10 repetitions with no rest in between. These exercises are often done in several sets for a push-and-pull movement or grouping a certain

Table 8-3.

Training Variables

- Plane of motion
- Speed of execution
- Range of motion
- Loading parameters (swiss balls, weight vest, dumbbells, tubing)
- Acute variables (sets, reps, tempo, duration)
- Body position
- Frequency
- Amount of control
- Amount of feedback

body part(s) performing the same set and repetition model.

- Split routine: Another great system for producing mass (hypertrophy). The routine consists of training chest/shoulders/triceps on 2 days (Monday and Thursday) of the week and back/biceps/legs on the other 2 days (Tuesday and Friday) with a 1-day break (Wednesday).

When designing strength training programs, it is important that the program be based on science. The program must be systematic, progressive, and functional. The program must incorporate principles of strength training mentioned previously to be effective. When performing strength training exercises, it is important to consult with a physician prior to beginning the program. A functional screen should be performed along with a body assessment (Table 8-3). Some examples of specific strength training exercises in an aquatic median are as follows:

A. Stabilization
1. Multiplanar step-up curl to press
2. Single-leg squat touch overhead press
3. Single-leg roman dead lift to overhead press
4. Single-leg rotation with Hydro-Tone (Hydro-Tone Fitness Systems, Inc, Orange, CA)
5. Skater's single-leg squat to overhead press
6. Base pulley with Hydro-Tone

B. Strength
1. Multiplanar lunge curl to press
2. Multiplanar lunge reach to row to press
3. Pitcher squat to press
4. Squat curl to press
5. Squat to shrug to calf raise
6. Base pulley Hydro-Tone

C. Power
1. Dumbbell snatch
2. Push press
3. Upper body

D. Stabilization
1. Single-leg Hydro-Tone press
2. Wall push-up with rotation
3. Hydro-Tone shoulder extension
4. Scaption
5. Cobra

E. Strength
1. Hydro-Tone press
2. Decline Hydro-Tone chest press
3. Front raise
4. Lateral raise
5. Biceps curls
6. Flyes
7. Hydro-Tone/dumbbell upright rows
8. Bent overrow

F. Power
1. Hydro-Tone chest pass against jets
2. Hydro-Tone rotational chest pass against jets
3. Single-leg Hydro-Tone chest pass
4. Lower body

G. Stabilization
1. Single-leg squats
2. Single-leg squats on box
3. Single-leg squats with touch down
4. Step-ups
5. Pitcher squats

H. Strength
1. Multiplanar lunge
2. Body weight squat
3. Multiplanar step-up
4. Posterior lunge
5. Elevated back lunge
6. Lateral lunge

I. Power
1. Tuck jumps
2. Squat jumps
3. Lunge jumps
4. Box jumps
5. Rotational jumps

CORE STABILIZATION

The core is where all movement begins; it is also where the center of gravity is located in the human body. In the previous chapter we noted that all functional movements should be multiplanar, requiring deceleration, stabilization, and acceleration. Knowing that these functional movements require such high complexity, quality muscular strength, and neuromuscular efficiency, the water provides a medium for which core training could be very beneficial.

The purpose of a core stability program is to improve dynamic postural control; assure proper muscular balance and joint arthrokinematics; and provide stability to the lumbar, pelvic, and hip region. This is the center/cornerstone of the body, where the majority of movements are produced and where the center of gravity is located. There are 29 muscles that attach to these regions. A core stability program that produces an efficient core will allow for quality length–tension relationships of all functional agonists and antagonists. The muscle groups within the core work as one functional unit. This enables the entire kinetic chain to work synergistically to produce force, reduce force, and stabilize against abnormal force. This is an area that needs to be trained appropriately to function efficiently.

In the past, very little time was put into the development of a proper core stabilization, strengthening, or power program. Most programs consisted of flexion and extension of the trunk region. There are no activities of daily living or sports that only require flexion and extension of the trunk region. Very few people develop the muscles that are required for spine stabilization.[3] The body's stabilization system must function very well to effectively utilize the strength, power, neuromuscular control, and muscular endurance that have been developed.

A properly designed core stabilization program will potentially help an individual with strength gains, muscular power, endurance gains, and neuromuscular control. Greater neuromuscular control along with adequate stabilizing strength will allow the kinetic chain to work in a more efficient position.

When talking about core training, it is important to understand the anatomy of the area. All the muscles shown in Table 8-2 play an important role due to how they stabilize the kinetic chain dynamically. These muscles work as a unit; individually each has a specific function and does not effectively stabilize alone.

When beginning a core training program it is important that stabilization has been achieved prior to strengthening and power exercises. It has been found that abdominal training without proper pelvic stabilization can increase intradiscal pressure and compressive forces in the lumbar spine.[17] It has also been found that hyperextension training without proper pelvic stabilization can cause intradiscal

Table 8-4.

Progression of Exercises

Slow ⟶ fast, simple ⟶ complex, low force ⟶ high force, stable ⟶ unstable surfaces, and increasing reps, sets, and intensities

pressures within the spine.[16] The muscles in the lumbar, pelvic, and hip complex that are considered the primary stabilizers are slow twitch muscles. These are muscles that respond best to time under tension. Core stabilization must be trained properly to allow an individual to maintain dynamic postural control for prolonged periods of time. As you begin core training there is something such as drawing in, which refers to the act of maximally activating the transverse abdominal musculature. To perform this action, you must stand erect and place your index finger on your umbilicus (belly button). Then you pull your belly button in toward your spine as far as possible using muscles, not by sucking in your breath. While performing this method it is important that you are able to continue to breathe normally. Another important method is maintaining cervical spine neutral positioning. Being in a neutral position with the cervical spine will keep the head from protracting, therefore decreasing compressive forces on C1 and providing more pelvic stability. During core training both of these methods will help improve posture, muscular balance, and stabilization.

A few guidelines should be addressed prior to performing core stabilization training and all other types of training as well. All individuals must undergo a thorough assessment or screening process by their physicians. All muscular imbalances and arthrokinematic deficits must be corrected prior to aggressive core training. All workouts should be progressive, systematic, and sport specific.

The programs should emphasize the basic stabilization principles for the entire muscular contraction (Phase I) followed by focusing on eccentric contractions, concentric contractions, and dynamic stabilization (Phase II). Core stability programs should be manipulated by changing variables such as plane of motion, range of motion, load parameters (physioballs, medicine balls, body blades, weight vest, dumb bells, tubing, Hydro-Tones, etc), body position, speed of excitation, amount of feedback, duration (sets, repetitions, tempo, time under tension), frequency, and weight depth.[4] All exercises must be safe, challenging, able to stress multiple planes, incorporate a multisensory environment, and derived from functional movement skills; that is, sports/activity-specific skills (Table 8-4). Using water as a medium to train provides those parameters, with a goal of developing optimal levels of functional strength and dynamic stabilization.

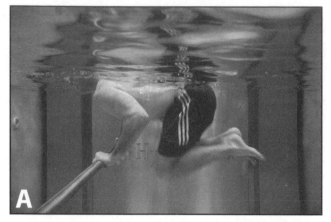

Figure 8-1. Knee to chest.

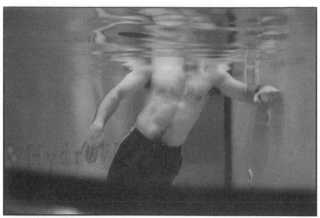

Figure 8-2. Static side bridge.

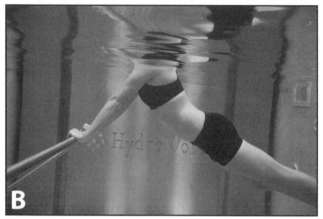

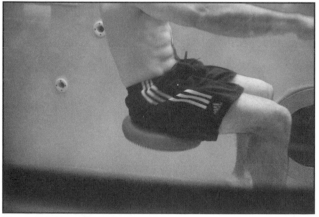

Figure 8-3. Dyna disc balance.

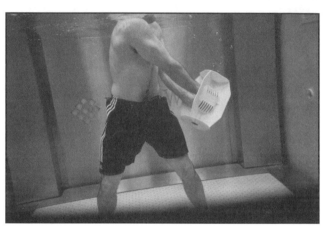

Figure 8-4. Wood chops.

4. Static stand against jets

5. Standing hip extension

6. Standing ball holds/balance

7. Swiss ball/DynaDisc (Exertools, Petaluma, CA) balance (Figure 8-3)

Core Stability Strength Training— Phase II

Exercises that incorporate dynamic concentric and eccentric activities through a full range of motion:

1. Wood chops—variations (Figure 8-4)

2. Ball crunch

3. Low abdominal crunches (Figures 8-5A and 8-5B)

4. Hydro-Tone rotation with resistance

5. Standing medicine ball kicks

6. Box patterns/figure 8s (Figure 8-6)

7. Step-up box bridge

Core Stability Training—Phase I

Exercises that involve little joint movement and are designed to improve intrinsic stabilization:

1. Core pulls

2. Knee to chest (all) with support bar (Figure 8-1)

3. Static side bridge (Figure 8-2)

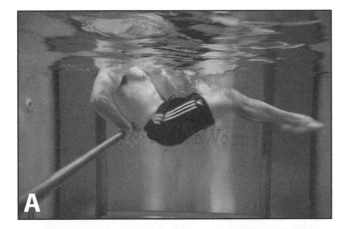

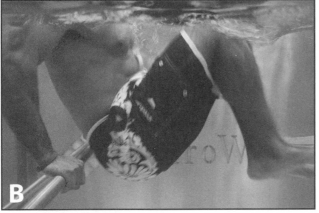

Figure 8-5. Low ab crunch.

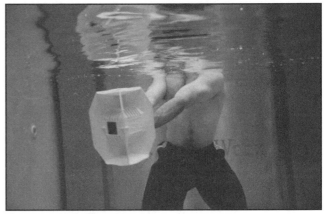

Figure 8-6. Hydro-Tone box pattern.

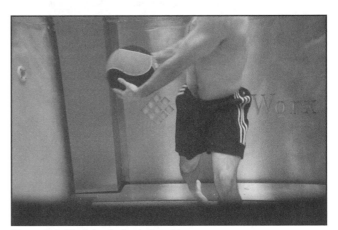

Figure 8-8. Medicine ball rotational toss.

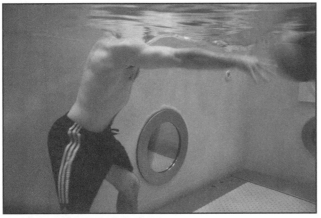

Figure 8-7. Medicine ball chest pass.

Core Stability Power Training

Exercises that are a combination of stability and strength that are sports specific and activity specific. These exercises are performed at an intensity, velocity, and speed that individuals will experience in their environment:

1. Hydro-Tone rotation with resistance

2. Hydro-Tone or medicine ball chest pass (Figure 8-7)

3. Hydro-Tone or medicine ball rotational toss (Figure 8-8)

4. Hydro-Tone or medicine ball oblique throw

CONCLUSION

A well-designed strength-training program will produce optimum levels of strength, neuromuscular control, power, flexibility, endurance, and changes to body composition. With proper physical conditioning for sports participation, the athlete should be prepared for high-level performance while decreasing the chance for injuries that are inherent to the particular sport. Having the opportunity to vary the training and training sessions to maximize athletic potential is critical in achieving peak performance.

REFERENCES

1. Kraemer WJ. Exercises prescription in weight training. A needs analysis. *NSCA J.* 1983;5:64–65.

2. Pearson D, Faigenbaum A, Conley M, Kraemer WJ. The NSCA basic guidelines for resistance training of athletes. *Strength Cond J.* 2000;22(4):14–27.

3. Baechle TR, Earle RW. *Essentials of Strength Training and Conditioning.* 3rd ed. Champaign, IL: Human Kinetics; 2008.

4. Martel GF, Harmer ML, Logan JM, Parker CB. Aquatic plyometric training increases vertical jump in female volleyball players. *Med Sci Sports Exerc.* 2005;37:1814–1819.

5. Robinson LE, Devor ST, Merrick MA, Buckworth J. The effects of land vs. aquatic plyometrics on power, torque, velocity, and muscle soreness in women. *J Strength Cond Res.* 2004;18:84–91.

6. Garhammer J. A review of power output studies of Olympic and power lifting: methodology, performance prediction, and evaluation tests. *J Strength Cond Res.* 1993;7(2):76–89.

7. Faulkner JA, Claflin DR, McCully KK. Power output of fast and slow fibers from human skeletal muscle. In: Jones NL, McCartney N, McComas AJ, eds. *Human Muscle Power.* Champaign, IL: Human Kinetics; 1986.

8. Hakkinen K, Hakkinen A. Neuromuscular adaptations during intensive strength training in middle-aged and elderly males and females. *Electromyogr Clin Neurophysiol.* 1995;35:137–147.

9. Marx JO. The effect of periodization and volume of resistance training in women [abstract]. *Med Sci Sports Exerc.* 1998;30(suppl 5):164.

10. Stone MH. Implications for connective tissue and bone alterations resulting from resistance exercise training. *Med Sci Sports Exerc.* 1988;20(suppl 5):162–168.

11. Lemon PW. Effects of exercise on dietary protein requirements. *Int J Sport Nutr.* 1998;8:426–447.

12. McLester JR, Bishop P, Guilliams ME. Comparison of 1 day and 3 days per week of equal-volume resistance training in experienced subjects. *J Strength Cond Res.* 2000;14:273–281.

13. Taaffe DR, Duret C, Wheeler S, Marcus R. Once-weekly resis¬tance exercise improves muscle strength and neuromuscular per-formance in older adults. *J Am Geriatr Soc.* 1999;47:1208–1214.

14. Stone MH, O'Bryant H, Garhammer J. A hypothetical model for strength training. *J Sports Med Phys Fitness.* 1981;21:342–351

15. Kraemer WJ, Stone MH, O'Bryant HS, et al. Effects of single vs. multiple sets of weight training: impact of volume, intensity, and variation. *J Strength Cond Res.* 1997;11:143–147.

16. Boyle M. *Functional Training for Sports.* Champaign, IL: Human Kinetics; 2004.

17. Bloomfield SA. Changes in musculoskeletal structure and func¬tion with prolonged bed rest. *Med Sci Sports Exerc.* 1997;29(2):197–206.

18. Hakkinen K, Alen M, Kallinen M, Newton RU, Kraemer WJ. Neuromuscular adaptation during prolonged strength training, detraining and re-strength-training in middle-aged and elderly people. *Eur J Appl Physiol.* 2000;83:51–62.

19. Fleck SJ, Kreamer WJ. *Designing Resistance Training Program.* 2nd ed. Champaign, IL: Human Kinetics; 1997.

Sports-Specific Training

Murphy Grant, MS, ATC, NASM-PES, CES

One of the main objectives of training is to systematically achieve improved physical, physiological, and performance adaptations. It is important to know the physiological demands of an activity or sport prior to designing a performance enhancement training program. The more specific the training is to the activity or sport, the greater the transfer of training effect.[1] Reproducing activity and movement in the training phase allows one to become more efficient during sports-specific activity.

PERIODIZATION TRAINING

Optimizing peak performance involves year-round training, which consists of many different training variables, as noted in the sections on plyometrics, core training, balance training, and strength training. All of these should be done when working to maximize athletic potential. But the intensity, volume, and structure should be different during preseason, in-season, and off-season.

Each sport requires different training variables for which success is the desired outcome. Periodization is an approach to conditioning that brings about peak performance while reducing the chance of injuries and overtraining in the athlete; involves organizing the training regimen into cycles of objectives, tasks, and content; and involves varying the variables of training, which include exercise mode, intensity, duration, and frequency.

Periodization is broken down into cycles. The overall or complete training session is referred to as a macrocycle.

This could be a single season or as long as 4 years for an Olympian. When designing programs, the periodization method is a good way to break down such specifics as when to change, utilize, and incorporate new ideas and exercises throughout a macrocycle.

Knowing the demands of each sport or position is necessary when designing an effective training and conditioning program. Knowing what training phase an athlete is in, and the goals associated with each phase, allows for quality and efficient workouts. A few key terms or training variables that must be understood include repetitions, sets, training intensity, training volume, exercise selection, exercise order, training duration, training frequency, and neural demands. For example, repetitions refers to the number of times an exercise movement is completed and depends on the work capacity and the intensity of exercises in the training phase.[2] There is an inverse relationship between exercise intensity and repetitions. A greater number of repetitions is associated with muscular endurance, whereas a lower number is associated with strength and power. Certain repetition ranges often yield training adaptations (Table 9-1). A set of exercises is the group of consecutive repetitions performed. As with repetitions, the number of sets will often yield training adaptations (Table 9-2). Training intensity is believed to be the most important training variable to consider when designing a program. It is the level of effort that an individual performs. Intensity is often determined by the number of sets and repetitions that need to be performed. Training in an unstable environment increases the training intensity; training in a multidimensional/multiplanar

Wilk KE, Joyner DM. *The Use of Aquatics in Orthopedic and Sports Medicine Rehabilitation and Physical Conditioning (pp 103-111).*
© 2014 SLACK Incorporated.

Table 9-1.

Types of Strength

Limit	The maximal amount of force that can be produced in a single contraction
Maximal strength	Maximum force a specific muscle in one effort can produce
Relative strength	The maximum force an individual can produce per unit of body weight
Endurance strength	Force that is produced and maintained over a period of time
Speed strength	Production of the most force that can be generated in the shortest possible time
Reactive strength	The ability of neuromuscular system to switch from eccentric contraction to a concentric contraction
Stabilizing strength	The strength of the muscles that involve the kinetic chain and stabilizing dynamic joint stabilization
Core strength	Muscle surrounding the area of the lumbar, pelvic, and hip region controlling the center of gravity
Functional strength	The production of multiplanar strength efficiency during functional movements

Table 9-3.

Guidelines for Strength Training

- General and medical history
- Sport/position
- Occupation
- Medication
- Lifestyle

environment will increase intensity. Increasing intensity will yield training adaptations (Table 9-3). The training volume is the total amount of work performed or weight that is lifted within a time period or workout session. Training volume is something that is high during early phases of a periodization regimen and then tapers off during the latter phases of a periodization regimen. Training volumes will vary among individuals and are based on goals, age, work capacity, and nutritional status. Training duration is the time needed or used from the beginning of a workout to competition. Most often, workouts lasting longer than 90 min will result in a decrease in form, stabilization, and energy levels. Finally, the training frequency is the number

Table 9-2.

Training Systems

• Single set	• Circuit training
• Multiple sets	• Peripheral heart action
• Pyramid	• Tri-set
• Super set	• Split routine

of sessions per week or per body part. Most often this is determined by the athlete's goals.

The selection of exercises has a great impact on the outcome of the training program. Other variables in an exercise program may not be able to compensate for improper exercises. The goals that have been set will have a large impact on the exercises that have been selected. It is important to understand what muscle groups will need to be trained, what motor patterns need to be addressed, and what energy systems are utilized in sports and in training programs. A sound analysis of the movements involved in a sport should be performed because this will help in the development of a safe and quality training program.

Exercise order is important in determining training responses. Exercises that are often placed early in a workout order are typically structural and power exercises that maximize strength and power. Strength and power exercises require more precise exercise form and technique and require higher energy levels. These exercises are often done for larger muscle groups. Exercises placed later in workouts may not be performed at the same intensity level. Power should be incorporated after a good strength base has been established. It is important that stabilization be established before strengthening.

Neural demands of training will help improved neuromuscular efficiency. This is done by progressively changing the body part in a plane of motion or by changing the base of support.

OFF-SEASON TRAINING

Periodization starts with off-season training, followed by preseason and in-season training, and ends with a transitional period. Off-season training is typically very structured and typically lasts 8 to 12 weeks or longer. It is also a preparatory period, a time to make gains physically and mentally without the stress of upcoming competitions. The preparatory phase includes a hypertrophy phase and endurance phase in which there is low-intensity and high-volume activity. The goal is to first develop a base of endurance followed by a strength base in which greater intensity training can occur. During the strength phase, intensity increases, some sports-specific activity is done, and there is a decrease in training volume.

Off-season training is followed by preseason training, which also typically lasts 8 to 12 weeks or longer. Preseason activities will consist of power activities, which are a combination of both strength and speed. The training that takes place will be at a very high intensity and at a level near competition. Volume is often decreased here to allow the body to recover.

In-season training will vary in duration, from a few weeks to a few months. Some periods of competitions only last 1 to 2 weeks. Other sports have the potential to last for several months. Knowing the demands of each sport and the individual participating in the activity will play a big role in the type of training activity. It is important during this time that the individual is in peak performance on days of competition. Intensity should be high during this time; volume should be low to moderate, while maintaining the strength and power that was gained during the off-season. Proper physical conditioning for sport activities should prepare the individual or athlete to perform at a high level while helping to prevent injuries.

Transitional training is a period of active rest. During this period, the athlete stays active but rests from the sport and sport-related movements that the athlete performs during the in-season period. This allows the body's tissues, which are highly stressed during the season, to rest and recover. The transition phase typically lasts for a few weeks.

When beginning sports-specific training, it is first essential to enhance the fundamentals of the skill. Sports-specific training then follows to enhance performance. High levels of strength and sports-specific training are prerequisites to superior speed, power, strength, endurance, and overall sporting performance. The principle of specificity states that training should mirror the demands of the sport as closely as possible.[3] This applies not only to the way the body's energy systems and neuromuscular system are taxed through manipulation of intensity and rest intervals but also to the movement patterns of each exercise.

Athletes should train movements rather than muscles. A simple example is the vertical jump. The muscles involved in the vertical jump—the calves, quadriceps, hamstrings, and gluteals—can be trained individually with exercise choices such as toe raises, leg extensions, leg curls, and kickbacks. A more appropriate exercise is a barbell squat, which closely matches the movement pattern of the vertical jump. Moreover, jump squats are even more specific to jumping and increase vertical jump performance to a greater extent than multi-muscle, multi-joint exercises such as the barbell squat or single-muscle, single-joint exercises such as the toe raise, leg extension, or leg curls. Athletes must be able to divide their time and energy among various types of training—endurance, strength and power, speed and agility, tactical, etc—as well as allow adequate time to

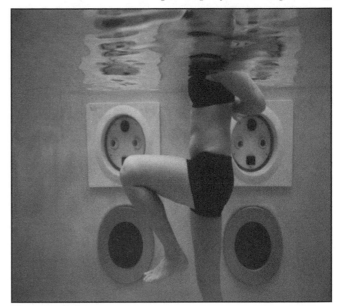

Figure 9-1. A-Skip.

recover so that overtraining does not occur. Sports-specific training for select sports will now be discussed.

BASEBALL

The game of baseball, "America's pasttime," requires skill, agility, speed, and coordination, as well as adequate range of motion and muscular strength, power, and endurance. Baseball demands an average time of 4.3 to 4.4 sec from home plate to first base and the ability to hit or throw a baseball with velocities in excess of 90 mph.

When preparing for the game of baseball, individuals should begin with a functional dynamic warm-up, with exercises such as A-Skip (Figure 9-1), knee hugs, walking lunge, lunge with twist, glute kicks, and more. Strength training should incorporate shoulder movements, trunk stability and rotation, and explosive power in the lower extremity, which can be done either on land or in the water. Sports-specific exercises that may be beneficial for those individuals training in an aquatic medium include the following:

- Decline press (Figure 9-2)
- Base pulley rows (Figure 9-3)
- Lateral raise (Figure 9-4)
- Posterior lunge (Figure 9-5)
- Shoulder extension (Figure 9-6)
- Wood chops (Figure 9-7)
- Single-leg box jumps (Figure 9-8)

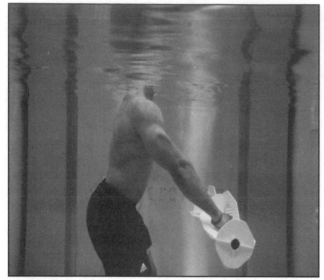

Figure 9-2. Decline press.

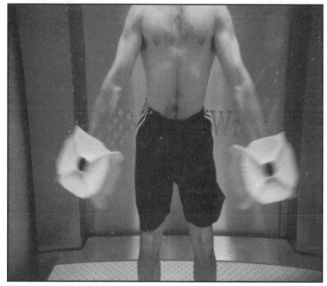

Figure 9-4. Lateral raise.

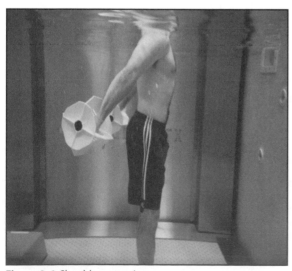

Figure 9-6. Shoulder extension.

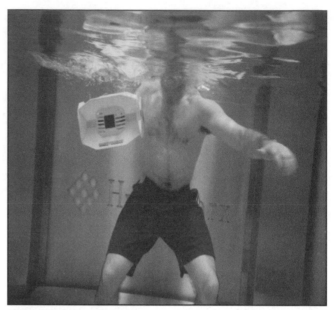

Figure 9-3. Base pulley rows.

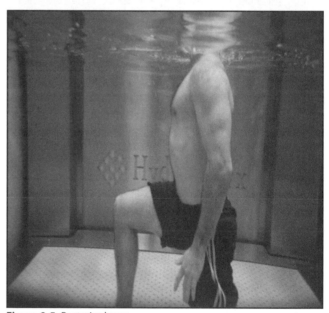

Figure 9-5. Posterior lunge.

BASKETBALL

Basketball is a sport that is popular among individuals at all age groups and skill levels. Basketball requires individuals to be strong, agile, and explosive while exhibiting fine motor skills when shooting and dribbling. The needs and demands of basketball are speed endurance, agility, speed, strength, and explosive power. These athletes need to jump to get a rebound and the agility to move into the low post to receive a pass and score. When preparing for the game of basketball, individuals should begin with a functional dynamic warm-up, with exercises such as A-Skip (see Figure 9-1), knee hugs, walking lunge, lunge with twist, glute kicks, and more. Sports-specific exercises that may

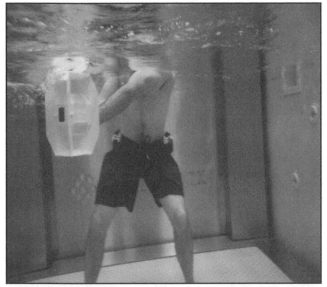

Figure 9-7. Wood chops.

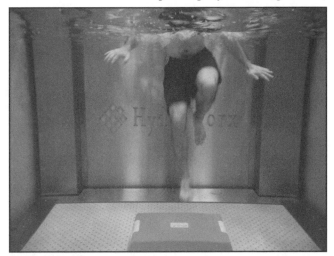

Figure 9-8. Single-leg box jumps.

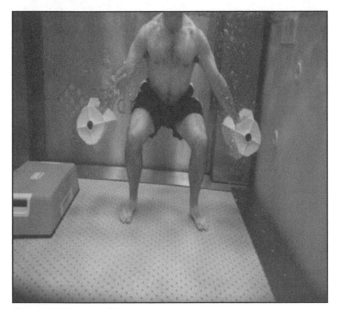

Figure 9-9. Squat curl to press.

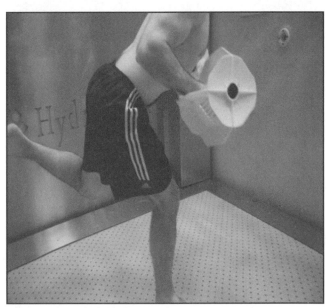

Figure 9-10. Single-leg balance and row.

be beneficial for those individuals training in an aquatic medium include the following:

- Squat curl to press (Figure 9-9)
- Single-leg balance and row (Figure 9-10)
- Power skip (Figure 9-11)
- Run and lateral shuffle (Figure 9-12)

SOCCER

Soccer is one of the most demanding sports. Few sports are played on such a large playing field and last as long without regular rest periods. Less than 2% of the total distance covered during a game is with the ball.[4] There are between 1000 and 12,000 bouts of dynamic change of direction.[4] The average sprint is roughly 15 m. Standing makes up roughly 17% of total activity, walking 24%, jogging 36%, and sprinting 8%. During a match these athletes will run approximately 10 km.

Exercises for sports-specific training must consist of balance, explosive power, muscular and speed endurance, and strength training.

Sports-specific exercises that may be beneficial for those individuals training in an aquatic medium include the following:

- Leg action (Figure 9-13)
- Ice skater (Figure 9-14)
- Multiplanar box jumps (Figure 9-15)
- Single-leg rotation (Figure 9-16)
- Single-leg squat on a box (Figure 9-17)

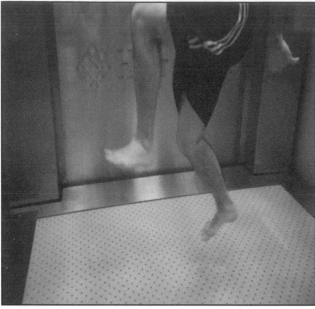

Figure 9-11. Power skip.

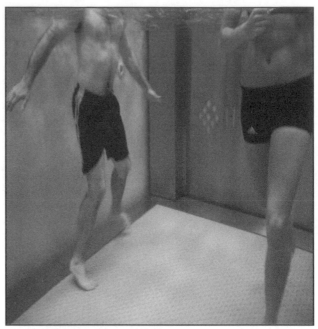

Figure 9-12. Run and lateral shuffle.

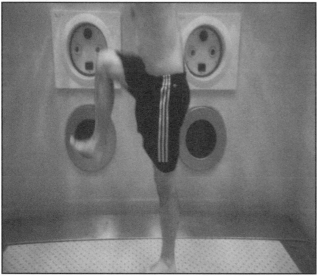

Figure 9-13. Leg action.

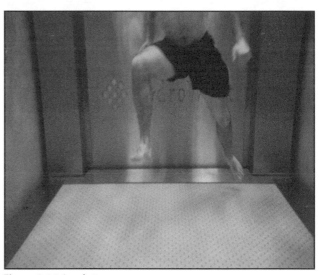

Figure 9-14. Ice skater.

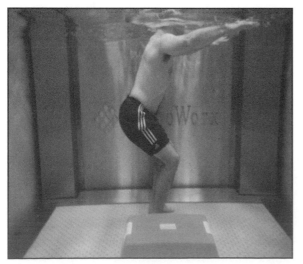

Figure 9-15. Multiplanar box jumps.

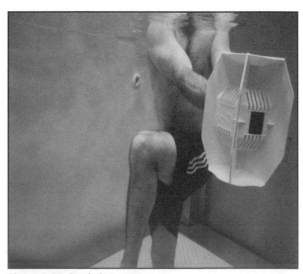

Figure 9-16. Single-leg rotation.

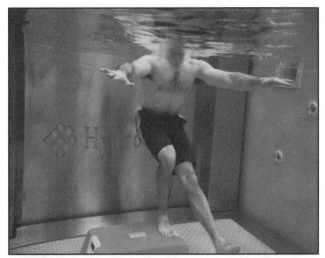

Figure 9-17. Single-leg squat on a box.

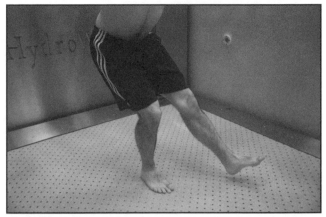

Figure 9-18. Balance and reach.

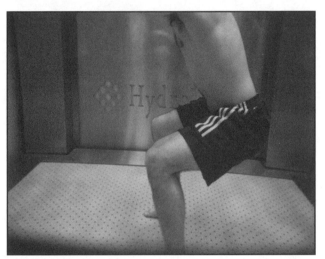

Figure 9-19. Body weight squat.

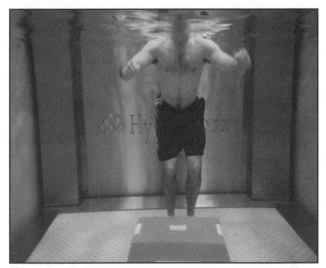

Figure 9-20. Box jump.

VOLLEYBALL

Structured sports-specific training programs for volleyball can increase explosive power, vertical jump height, stamina, speed, and agility around the court. Volleyball is a game in which all of these attributes are necessary. Volleyball players have exceptional lower body power and perform very well in the vertical jump text.[3,4] Volleyball players move around the court methodically and efficiently, in order to get to areas on the court to make plays. Power in the hips and thighs is necessary to jump explosively off the ground in order to spike, set, and dive. Stability in the core and lower body is also important for performance as well as in reducing injury risk.

The repetitive nature of jumping movements makes strength, power, and endurance important aspects of training.[4] Strength and power may be more important than aerobic endurance in the game of volleyball, although elite-level volleyball players typically have moderate to high levels of aerobic power.[3,4]

Exercises for sports-specific training must consist of agility, speed, explosive power, balance, and absolute strength. Sports-specific exercises that may be beneficial for those individuals training in an aquatic medium include the following:

- Balance and reach (Figure 9-18)
- Body weight squat (Figure 9-19)
- Box jump (Figure 9-20)
- Depth jump (Figure 9-21)
- Ice skater (Figure 9-22)
- Lateral jump (Figure 9-23)
- Lunge jump (Figure 9-24)
- Multiplanar box jump (see Figure 9-15)
- Run and lateral shuffle (see Figure 9-12)
- Single-leg hop (Figure 9-25)
- Squat jump (Figure 9-26)

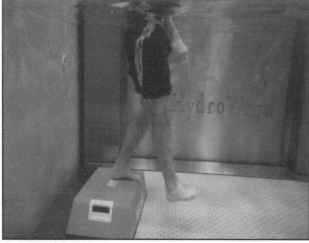

Figure 9-21. Depth jump.

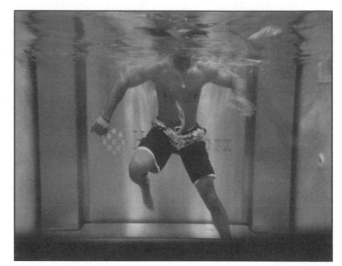

Figure 9-22. Ice skater.

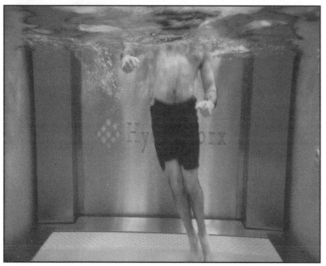

Figure 9-23. Lateral jump.

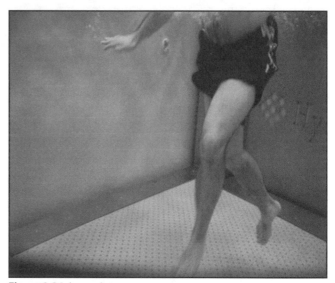

Figure 9-24. Lunge jump.

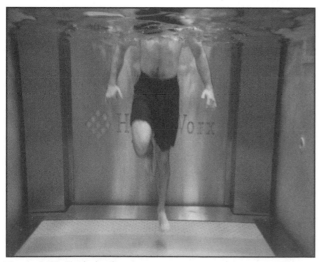

Figure 9-25. Single-leg hop.

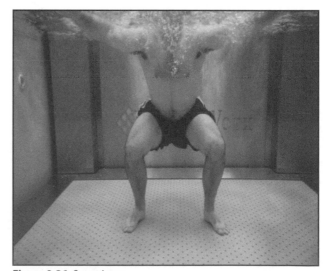

Figure 9-26. Squat jump.

CONCLUSION

A well designed sports-specific training program will produce optimum levels of strength, neuromuscular control, power, flexibility, endurance, and changes to body composition. With proper physical conditioning for sports participation, the athlete should be prepared for high-level performance while decreasing the chance for injuries that are inherent to the particular sport. Having the opportunity to vary the training and training sessions to maximize athletic potential is critical in achieving peak performance.

REFERENCES

1. Hakkinen K. Neuromuscular adaption during strength training. Aging, detraining and immobilization. *Crit Rev Phys Rehab Med.* 1994;6:161-198.
2. Tan B. Manipulating resistance training program variables to optimize maximum strength in men: a review. *J Strength Cond Res.* 1999;13:289-304.
3. Rutherford OM, Jones DA. The role of learning and coordination in strength training. *Eur J Appl Physiol.* 1986;55:100-105.
4. Clark M. NASM optimal performance training for the performance enhancement specialist. *Performance Profile.* 2004;4:197-204.

Section IV

Research and Evidence

10

Research Evidence for the Benefits of Aquatic Exercise

Stephen F. Crouse, PhD, FACSM and Dennis Dolny, PhD

Regular physical exercise is widely recognized for its health benefits. Professional organizations concerned with health and disease prevention, such as the American Heart Association and the American College of Sports Medicine (ACSM), universally encourage children and adults to take appropriate exercise each day.[1] There is substantial evidence that doing so will lower the risk of heart disease and cancer, increase bone density, improve muscle strength, boost physical working capacity, and augment mental alertness regardless of age.

The current recommendations for healthy exercise include at minimum (1) vigorous or moderate intensity aerobic activity performed 20 min a day twice a week to 30 min a day 5 days a week and (2) strength training exercises for the major muscle groups of the body at least twice a week.[1,2] Unfortunately, for many Americans these exercise goals are unattainable due to physical limitations that may result, for example, from injury or surgery, osteoarthritis, obesity, or diminished strength due to aging. A low-impact, nonweight-bearing form of exercise is recommended for individuals with these types of limitations.[2] In this regard, aquatic exercise may prove beneficial because it is associated with a significant reduction in the repetitive stress and strain on the lower extremities and spine that is typical of land-based activities.[3,4]

It is also this reduction of foot-striking forces in the aquatic medium compared to land-based ambulation that makes this an attractive mode of exercise for athletes, those most physically fit in our society. Athletes suffering from overuse injuries or injuries resulting from participation in their chosen sport require an alternate exercise mode to limit detraining during rehabilitation. In addition, athletes practice various cross-training strategies throughout their training year to optimize the training stimulus and further improve performance. Thus, athletes may engage in aquatic exercise for conditioning benefits, either while recovering from an injury or to introduce a cross-training stimulus.

Non-swimming aquatic exercise has increased in popularity in recent years.[5] In addition to swimming, aquatic exercise forms include water aerobics, deep water running (DWR), shallow water running (SWR), and cycle ergometry. Recently, a relatively new type of aquatic exercise equipment, an aquatic treadmill (ATM), has been developed that joins a variable-speed underwater treadmill with pump-driven directional water jets to provide frontal resistance to ambulation through the water. This system emulates the exercise intensity control enabled by land treadmill (LTM) velocity and grade adjustments, permitting the user to engage in familiar walking and running activities and vary the intensity by increasing the treadmill velocity and changing the resistive force of the water jets. It is our purpose in this chapter to provide the reader with research related to the effectiveness of aquatic exercise for physical training and health benefits, with a particular focus on the recent findings using the ATM.

Wilk KE, Joyner DM. *The Use of Aquatics in Orthopedic and Sports Medicine Rehabilitation and Physical Conditioning (pp 115-128).*

BRIEF REVIEW OF AQUATIC EXERCISE LITERATURE

Compared to the extensive literature that documents the physiologic responses to various forms of land exercise, few studies have been published to characterize the physiologic and training effects of nonswimming aquatic exercise. In this short review, we will provide a summary of what is known about the effectiveness of various aquatic head-out exercise modes of training to improve physical fitness, particularly focusing on cardiovascular fitness. We will also document to the extent possible the physiologic responses that have been found when one performs aquatic exercise compared to performing traditional land-based exercise. For more extensive reviews, the interested reader is referred to Barbosa et al[6] and Reilly et al.[7]

AQUATIC AEROBICS EXERCISE AND CYCLING

Aquatic aerobics and dance are very popular modes of exercise, whereas water cycling is less frequently employed in exercise settings. DWR and SWR are also popular aquatic exercise modes that will be reviewed later in this chapter. A limited number of studies exist to quantify the acute and training responses to aquatic aerobics and cycling modes. Published studies generally support the effectiveness of these exercise types to produce a physiologic challenge to the cardiorespiratory and musculoskeletal system consistent with endurance training recommendations published by the ACSM[2] and can improve physical fitness.

Relatively few papers have been published to characterize the physiologic or training responses to head-out water cycling exercise. Frangolias and Rhodes[4] reported in their literature review that when comparing land to water cycle ergometry, no differences were found in measured maximum oxygen consumption (VO_{2max}) values, but heart rate (HR) at maximal exertion was typically lower in water cycling exercise. Sheldahl et al[8] reported that head-out water immersion resulted in a cephalad shift in blood volume at rest and an increase in left ventricular end diastolic dimension during aquatic cycling compared to land exercise. In a study on adult men, these researchers found that 12 weeks of aquatic cycle exercise training produced similar increases in VO_{2max} and submaximal stroke volume, accompanied by decreases in blood pressure and HR at submaximal work intensities. These results support the conclusion that the cardiovascular adaptation to cycle ergometer exercise in water is equivalent to that on land, despite resting differences in some cardiovascular parameters.

Compared to water cycling, more research has been published to characterize water aerobic exercise and the training responses that accrue when this form of exercise is chronically employed. The acute cardiorespiratory and metabolic responses depend on several factors, including the water depth, number of body segments in action, frequency of limb movement, and, for music-accompanied aerobics, the music cadence.[6] These various factors affecting the physiologic and metabolic responses make comparisons among studies difficult to interpret. For example, Benelli et al[9] reported that women performing identical aerobics exercise routines on land, in shallow water (0.8 m), and in deep water (1.4 m) showed progressively lower HRs (162, 154, and 113 bpm, respectively) and blood lactates (5.65, 3.15, and 1.75 mmoL/L, respectively). Based on the HR data, they concluded that exercise in water reduces the intensity of the aerobic exercise, and this intensity reduction is a function of the water depth. Evans and Cureton[10] further reported that bench-stepping exercise in water resulted in a lower VO_2 and rating of perceived exertion compared to performing the same bench-stepping exercise on land. This is not surprising because the step exercise was performed in chest-deep water, where the buoyant force of the water greatly reduced the gravitational resistive force, resulting in less energy requirement compared to land. However, the findings of Darby and Yaekle[11] suggest that a lower HR in water cannot necessarily be interpreted as a lower oxygen and energy requirement. These researchers reported that adding arms to leg exercise in water increased HR and oxygen uptake. More interesting, they measured oxygen uptake during water and land exercise and found that oxygen uptake was 2 to 6 mL $O_2 \cdot kg^{-1} \cdot min^{-1}$ higher during water exercise compared to land exercise performed at any equivalent submaximal HR. Subsequent regression analysis of their HR–oxygen uptake data demonstrated a shift to the right for water compared to land exercise. Their results applied to the ACSM prescription template for aerobic conditioning[2] demonstrated that any desired training HR during upright water aerobic exercise should be decreased about 7 to 13 bpm compared to HRs on land to attain an oxygen uptake intensity equivalent to land exercise. From these studies, it can be concluded that performing identical exercise movements in water will generally result in a comparatively lower HR than equivalent exercise on land. However, prescribing exercise in water based on traditional HR–VO_2 relationships derived on land may lead to errors in the exercise intensity. Specific HR–VO_2 relationships should be derived for water exercise and applied to exercise prescription practices.

Aerobic movements in water used in physical training programs that conform to the ACSM guidelines for exercise prescription[2] generally result in improvements in physical fitness that are at least comparable to training on land.[6] Women subjects, especially postmenopausal women, comprise most of the subjects in published studies, and comparable studies in men are lacking. Bocalini et al[12] and Takeshima et al[13] reported that aquatic exercise performed by older women 3 times per week, 60 to 70 min per session at 50% to 85% of maximal HR intensity for 12 weeks resulted in a 12% to 42% improvement in VO_{2max} and a 10% reduction in resting HR. These cardiorespiratory fitness benefits were comparable to those found when women performed equivalent exercise on land. Added physical fitness benefits of water exercise training reported by these researchers were significant improvements in measures of shoulder, back, leg, and chest strength (+6% to 13%), as well as gains in trunk flexibility (+50%) and in a chair stand test (+54%). Others have shown that adding aquatic resistance movements to the water exercise repertoire can produce gains in muscular strength in women at least as great as those achieved using elastic bands on land.[14] Moreover, in response to various modes and months of aquatic aerobic training, total cholesterol, low-density lipoprotein cholesterol, and body fat were reportedly reduced.[13,14] Aquatic exercise therapy has also been successfully applied to patients in cardiopulmonary rehabilitation programs, resulting in significant improvements in aerobic capacity (+12%) and strength (+13%), accompanied by reductions in sum of skinfolds used as a measure of body fat (−4.3 mm), total cholesterol (−4.4%), and triglycerides (−10.2%).[15] Therapeutic benefits of water exercise equal to and exceeding those from comparable land exercise have also been documented in patients with chronic obstructive pulmonary disease.[16] The summary of the literature suggests that aquatic exercise has proven physical fitness and health benefits, at least in older women and some patient populations, though more research is needed in adult men.

HEAD-OUT DEEP WATER RUNNING

DWR has become popular as an adjunct to land-based running and rehabilitation exercises, due in part to its potential to reduce repetitive strain and stress to the lower extremities. Participants typically run in an indoor pool in neck-deep water for DWR and may incorporate flotation/resistance devices about the waist, feet, and hands to help maintain posture and add to the workload of the activity.

Acute Physiological and Biomechanical Response to Deep Water Running

DWR has been studied by evaluating both the acute and chronic physiological effects. The majority of studies have demonstrated that DWR produces a lower peak oxygen consumption (VO_{2max} or VO_{2peak}) and HR compared to treadmill exercise on land.[17–24] Maximal effort exercise VO_2 and HR during DWR were approximately 86.5% and 90.4% of maximal LTM exercise responses, respectively.[7] Several factors may account for this difference, including

water's hydrostatic effect of increasing thoracic pressure, resulting in a lower HR during DWR, plus methodological factors such as short exercise test durations, changes in the kinematic characteristics of the DWR technique, and subjects' self-selected exercise intensity.[7]

Due to the lack of a ground support phase during DWR exercise, there is the potential for DWR to be performed with a variety of lower extremity patterns, such as incorporating either a high knee (HK), in which the legs move in a piston-like pattern, or cross-country (CC), where the stride pattern attempts to duplicate a land-running pattern. These different styles of leg movement patterns likely influence cardiorespiratory and neuromuscular factors. For example, Killgore et al[25] compared HK and CC DWR styles with LTM running at similar rates of VO_2 and reported a significantly lower stride rate for CC (54 strides·min^{-1}) versus HK (69 strides·min^{-1}) versus LTM running (80 strides·min^{-1}). CC was more like LTM running relative to the overall range of motion (ROM) of the gait pattern and thus possibly satisfied the specificity of training principle, yet HK was more like LTM running with regards to stride rate. Knee hyperextension was also present during CC and practitioners were cautioned to limit the full extension of the leg.

Kilding et al[26] compared LTM running with DWR where subjects were instructed to use their normal land-running actions at slow (72 cycles·min^{-1}) and fast (92 cycles·min^{-1}) cadences. Hip ROM was greater for DWR due to a combination of less flexion with much greater extension than in LTM running. Of greater importance was the observation that the knee and hip moved in a synchronized pattern (flexing or extending simultaneously) with no time lag between knee and hip movement initiation. This contrasts with LTM running, where a pattern of knee flexion/hip extension and knee extension/hip flexion with a significant time lag (hip joint movement prior to knee joint movement) occurs on land.

Deep Water Running Exercise Training Studies

The majority of research involving DWR training originally focused on the ability of DWR to maintain subjects' fitness levels following an initial training period of land running (see Reilly et al[7] for a review). With few exceptions, DWR has been effective in retaining the aerobic capacity (VO_{2max}) of participants who had previously trained on land. In previously untrained subjects, Reilly et al[27] determined that training with DWR was equally effective as LTM running and a combination of DWR and LTM running for improving VO_{2max} on an LTM and VO_{2peak} during DWR. However, the specificity principle was demonstrated whereby the group that trained using LTM running or DWR demonstrated a greater gain in aerobic capacity during that mode of testing. Meredith-Jones et al[28] combined DWR interspersed with resistance exercises for 12 weeks and reported significant increases in VO_{2peak} (10%) and muscular strength (32%) and decreased waist circumference (5%) in older (mean age = 59 years), overweight (body mass index [BMI] = 33 kg·m^2) women. Broman et al[29] reported that VO_{2max} increased 10% in elderly (mean age = 69 years) women following 8 weeks of interval-style DWR. DWR has also been used effectively with patients diagnosed with fibromyalgia[30] to improve peak aerobic capacity and emotional well-being in sedentary women.

Due to the lack of an ability to set a specific workload during DWR, it appears that the ability to regulate exercise intensity during DWR may be a confounding factor in determining the relative effectiveness of DWR to improve aerobic capacity. Using both HR and rate of perceived exertion to facilitate subjects' self-selected exercise intensity is recommended, with the acknowledgement that maximum HR during DWR is approximately 10% lower than during LTM running and should be accounted for when establishing a DWR exercise prescription.

Deep Water Running and Muscle Recruitment Patterns

Kaneda et al[31] reported muscle recruitment patterns (electromyography, EMG) of 6 lower extremity muscles during self-selected low, moderate, and high intensities of DWR and water and land walking. During DWR, soleus and gastrocnemius EMG were lower and biceps femoris was higher compared to land and water walking. Water buoyancy likely was responsible for lower soleus and gastrocnemius activities during DWR, and the greater biceps femoris activity was a result of greater degree of knee flexion and hip extension compared to land and water walking. Rectus femoris EMG was greater for DWR and water walking versus land walking, suggesting that DWR stimulates flexors and extensors of the hip while reductions in vertical loads reduce ankle plantarflexion muscle activity.[32] Finally, Kaneda et al[33] investigated the EMG activity of selected hip and trunk muscles during DWR compared to water walking. During DWR, adductor longus and gluteus medius EMG activity was greater than that of water and land walking, likely due to the greater hip ROM in DWR compared to water and land walking. EMG activity of erector spinae, rectus abdominus, and obliquus externus abdominis were all greater during DWR than during water and land walking due to a greater forward inclination and unstable floating condition.

HEALTH-RELATED AND THERAPEUTIC BENEFITS OF AQUATIC TREADMILL EXERCISE IN PREVIOUSLY UNTRAINED INDIVIDUALS

As reviewed previously, the physiologic responses and training benefits to several modes of aquatic exercise, DWR and SWR, and aquatic cycle ergometry have been documented in the literature. However, a precise, reproducible, and consistent exercise prescription is difficult to achieve because so many variables, which are not easily controlled, affect the physiologic responses.[6] In this regard, the recently developed variable-speed ATM system with adjustable water depth and frontal resistance provided by pump-driven directional water jets presents distinct advantages to more traditional modes of aquatic exercise. This system provides the benefit common to other aquatic exercise modes in that water buoyancy allows for an unloading effect during walking and jogging, thus reducing joint stress and consequent joint injury, especially in the obese and those recovering from joint injury or surgery. A second and distinct benefit is that the walking or running intensity can be precisely and reproducibly controlled through operator command over the treadmill velocity and jet resistance. A brief review of research using the ATM for fitness training follows here.

Quantifying Cardiovascular Responses to Aquatic Treadmill Exercise Compared to Land Treadmill Exercise

Few studies have been published to quantify the cardiovascular and physiologic responses to ATM-based exercise or to compare and contrast the responses with those measured during traditional LTM exercise. Existing studies are of mixed results, likely due to study differences in water depth; temperature; exercise protocols; and subject training status, health, and gender.

Greene et al[34] documented the oxygen cost and HR response of ATM exercise in chest-deep water with frontal jet resistance compared to equivalent treadmill velocity walking or jogging on an LTM. Twenty-four men and 25 women were studied to compare submaximal and

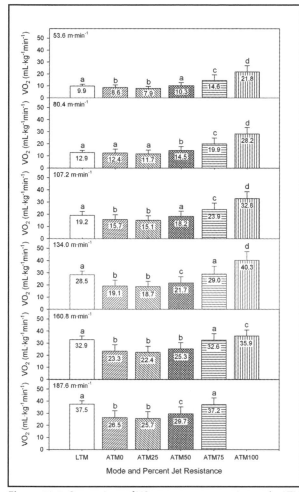

Figure 10-1. Comparison of VO_2 response to exercise on the LTM and ATM at varying jet resistance. Values are means $\pm$ SD. Data were analyzed using repeated measures analysis of variance, with comparisons among modes made with Duncan's multiple range test. Within each velocity, bars with different letters are significantly different (P < .05). (Reprinted with permission from Greene NP, Greene ES, Carbuhn AF, Green JS, Crouse SF. VO_2 prediction and cardiorespiratory responses during underwater treadmill exercise. *Res Q Exerc Sport.* 2011;82(2):264–273.)

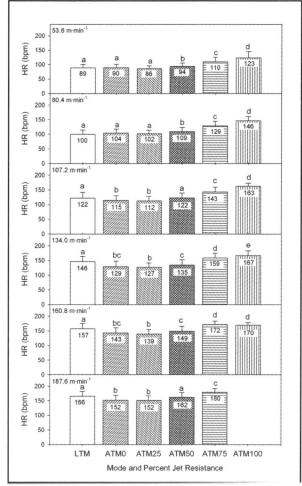

Figure 10-2. Comparison of HR response to exercise on the LTM and ATM at varying jet resistance. Values are means $\pm$ SD. Data were analyzed using repeated measures analysis of variance, with comparisons among modes made with Duncan's multiple range test. Within each velocity, bars with different letters are significantly different (P < .05). (Reprinted with permission from Greene NP, Greene ES, Carbuhn AF, Green JS, Crouse SF. VO_2 prediction and cardiorespiratory responses during underwater treadmill exercise. *Res Q Exerc Sport.* 2011;82(2):264–273.)

maximal cardiorespiratory responses between ATM and LTM exercise. The combined mean age, height, weight, and BMI was 41 years, 173.9 cm, 88.3 kg, and 29.0 kg·(m²)⁻¹, respectively. Each subject completed 6 separate experimental exercise sessions on 6 different days: (1) LTM at 0% grade; (2) ATM exercise at 0% jet (ATM0), (3) ATM exercise at 25% jet (ATM25), (4) ATM exercise at 50% jet (ATM50), (5) ATM exercise at 75% jet (ATM75), and (6) ATM exercise at 100% of maximal jet resistance (ATM100). Jet resistance was held constant at the prescribed percentage during the treadmill exercise on all exercise days. During each exercise session, the treadmill velocity was progressively increased in 3-min stages as follows: 53.6, 80.4, 107.2, 134.0, 160.8, and 187.6 m·min⁻¹. Oxygen uptake and HR were measured continuously throughout each exercise session until the exercise protocol was completed or the subject

reached voluntary exhaustion. The results for VO_2 and HR are shown in Figures 10-1 and 10-2. It is noteworthy that at any treadmill speed, with the exception of 80.4 m·min⁻¹, an ATM jet force of at least 50% was required to match or exceed LTM VO_2. At all treadmill velocities, LTM VO_2 exceeded ATM exercise with zero jet resistance. The HR data follow a similar trend. These data show that ATM exercise is less energy demanding than LTM running unless some additional resistance (in this case the water jets) provides a counterforce to forward ambulation. Interestingly, the VO_2 and HRs measured at 100% jet force in the ATM matched the corresponding LTM measures at a velocity 53.6 m·min⁻¹ faster.

Other related published studies are few and the results mixed. Fujishima and Shimizu[35] set LTM and ATM exercise intensity for elderly men at an equivalent rate of perceived exertion and found no significant differences in submaximal exercise VO_2 or HRs between the 2 exercise modes when no water jet resistance was employed, and the subjects in the ATM were submerged to the level of the xyphoid process. In contrast to these findings, Hall et al[36] reported a higher VO_2 and HR for rheumatoid arthritis patients submerged to the waist and walking (58.3 and 75 m·min^{-1}) on an ATM compared to the same velocity on an LTM. Dolbow et al[37] reported similar findings of comparatively higher VO_2 and HRs in response to ATM walking in waist-deep water by older (average age 58 years) men and women. Although the published literature is sparse, it is clear that results of ATM studies vary considerably. The variability is likely due to interstudy differences in such factors as the physical fitness status and age of the subjects; the depth of the water in the ATM; the exercise protocol, including the ambulation velocity and whether or not resistive jets were employed in the ATM system; and the water temperature.[6] It is important that practitioners and clinicians appreciate the factors that affect physiologic responses to submaximal ATM exercise so that they may account for them in their exercise prescriptions to ensure the safety of their patients and clients.

Maximal cardiorespiratory responses have also been measured, though rarely, in ATM exercise and compared to maximal responses derived from LTM exercise. Silvers et al[38] measured the cardiorespiratory responses of 23 college runners to maximal-effort exercise using an LTM and an ATM equipped with resistance jets. The subjects were exercised using an incremental protocol on the LTM and in the ATM submerged in 28°C water to the xyphoid process. In these trained men and women, maximal values measured during LTM running and ATM exercise for VO_2 (52.5 versus 52.8 mL·kg^{-1}·min^{-1}), HR (190 versus 189 bpm), and respiratory exchange ratio (1.17 versus 1.15) were not significantly different. Greene et al[34] confirmed the findings of equivalent VO_{2max} values during maximal-exertion exercise on an LTM and an ATM (30.1 versus 30.8 mL·kg^{-1}·min^{-1}) in older (age = 41 years), overweight (BMI = 29 kg·[m^2]$^{-1}$) men and women (n = 49). However, in contrast to the findings in younger trained men and women, both maximal HR (171 versus 167) and respiratory exchange ratio (1.20 versus 1.04) were significantly higher during maximal-effort LTM exercise by the older, untrained subjects.

Greene et al[34] were the first to develop 2 regression equations to estimate VO_2 during ATM exercise in a system with frontal resistance jets. As with the ACSM equations for estimating VO_2 during LTM and cycle ergometer exercise,[2] these new aquatic exercise equations will prove useful for practitioners in developing accurate exercise prescription intensities based on oxygen uptake for ATM exercise. Knowing VO_2 also enables the practitioner to estimate caloric expenditure during exercise, an important factor for prescribing exercise in weight management programs. The ACSM has published exercise intensity prescriptions

based on the application of percentage of maximal HR and HR reserve, yet these methods rely upon a linear HR–VO_2 relationship derived from exercise on land.[2] Greene et al[34] found that this relationship is linear during water-based exercise, but the regression coefficients (slope) differ from those derived from land-based treadmill exercise. Others have reported similar findings; that is, that HR is different at the same VO_2 in water compared to land exercise.[23,39] Thus, a regression to predict VO_2 that is derived from LTM exercise would not be valid to estimate VO_2 during ATM exercise. For ATM exercise with various jet settings, Greene et al[34] recommended the following:

1. For resistance jet settings from 0% to 25%:

Weight-relative VO_2 (mLO$_2$·kg^{-1}·min^{-1}) = 0.26144 × Height (cm) + 0.13482 × Velocity (m·min^{-1}) − 0.11966 × Weight (kg) − 33.72236

2. For resistance jet settings ≥25% through 100%:

Weight-relative VO_2 (mLO$_2$·kg^{-1}·min^{-1}) = 0.19248 × Height (cm) + 0.17422 × Jet Resistance (% max) + 0.14092 × Velocity (m·min^{-1}) − 0.12794 × Weight (kg) − 26.82489

Effectiveness of Aquatic Treadmill Exercise Training for Physical Fitness and Weight Reduction in Overweight and Obese Individuals

It is well accepted that obesity is a major risk factor for chronic disease morbidity and mortality and contributes to poor quality of life. Exercise and nutritional intervention are the primary measures employed in prevention and treatment.[1] However, traditional modes of exercise, such as walking or running, result in stress forces on the lower extremities that are accentuated in the obese and can lead to musculoskeletal injury and, as a result, discontinuance of exercise training.[40–42] Aquatic exercise is known to reduce the stress of exercise on the lower extremities and is a recommended mode of physical training for the obese and those with osteoarthritis.[43] Because exercise on an ATM with frontal jet resistance can induce acute cardiorespiratory and metabolic responses equivalent to those during LTM exercise, chronic training in this system would be hypothesized to have health benefits.

Greene et al[44] were the first to compare changes in physical fitness, body weight, and body composition in physically untrained, overweight, and obese adults (n = 57, average age = 44 years, weight = 90.5 kg, BMI = 30.5 kg·m^{-2}) after 12 weeks of LTM or ATM training. The subjects were randomly assigned to exercise 3 times per week for 12 weeks on either an LTM (n = 29) or an ATM (n = 28) with both groups matched for gender, intensity, and volume. Session volume was progressively increased from 250 to 500 kcal/session by week 6 and remained at 500 kcal through week 12. Caloric restriction diets were not imposed on the

Table 10-1.

Aerobic Fitness and Body Composition Changes Following Exercise Training

Variable	Land Treadmill		Aquatic Treadmill		P Value[a]
	Pretraining	Posttraining	Pretraining	Posttraining	
Maximal Aerobic Capacity					
VO_{2max} (L/min)	2.4±0.1	2.7±0.1	2.5±0.1	2.8±0.1	<.0001
VO_{2max} (mL O2·kg^{-1}·min^{-1})	27.29±1.19	31.24±1.31	26.91±1.22	30.17±1.24	<.0001
Body Mass and Girth Measurements					
Body mass (kg)	89.6±3.4	88.1±3.2	90.3±3.4	89.6±3.3	<.001
Body mass index (kg·m^{-2})	30.7±1.0	30.1±1.0	29.9±0.9	29.4±0.9	<.0001
Waist (cm)	97.5±3.3	93.7±3.0	96.8±2.3	93.2±2.0	<.0001
Hip (cm)	112.0±2.0	109.7±2.0	112.0±2.0	110.2±2.3	<.001
Waist : hip ratio	0.87±0.02	0.85±0.02	0.86±0.02	0.84±0.01	<.05
Total Body Composition					
Android % fat	43.8±2.2	42.3±2.1	45.7±1.2	44.3±1.4	<.01
Gynoid % fat	43.9±1.9	43.3±2.0	43.8±2.0	42.5±2.1	<.01
Android : gynoid ratio	1.03±0.06	1.02±0.06	1.09±0.05	1.09±0.05	NS
Lean body mass (kg)	51.2±2.2	51.1±2.1	51.9±2.4	52.5±2.4[b]	NS
Total fat mass (kg)	33.9±2.3	32.8±2.2	33.7±2.0	32.8±2.1	<.01
Regional Body Composition					
Arm % fat	34.0±2.0	33.4±2.0	32.3±2.0	31.4±2.2	<.01
Leg % fat	40.1±2.3	39.4±2.3	39.3±2.2	38.5±2.3	<.01
Trunk % fat	41.1±1.9	40.2±2.0	42.3±1.4	40.8±1.6	<.01
Regional Lean Mass					
Arm lean mass (kg)	5.6±0.4	5.6±0.4	5.9±0.4	6.0±0.4	NS
Trunk lean mass (kg)	24.9±5.9	24.5±5.1	25.2±6.1	25.0±5.9	NS
Regional Fat Mass					
Arm fat mass (kg)	2.8±0.2	2.7±0.2	2.7±0.2	2.7±0.2	NS
Leg fat mass (kg)	11.9±0.9	11.7±0.9	11.4±0.8	11.5±0.9	NS
Trunk fat mass (kg)	18.3±1.4	17.5±1.4	18.8±1.3	17.8±1.4	<.001

[a]Significance values reflect posttraining changes for both exercise training modes. Values are presented as means ±SE. NS indicates not significant.

[b]Total lean body mass increase approached significance with ATM training only (mode by training P=.0599).

Reprinted with permission from Greene NP, Lambert BS, Greene ES, Carbuhn AF, Green JS, Crouse SF. Comparative efficacy of water and land treadmill training for overweight or obese adults. *Med Sci Sports Exerc.* 2009;41:1808–1815.

subjects. Before and after training, VO_{2max} was assessed by means of an LTM protocol[45] with open-circuit calorimetry, and body composition was measured by dual-energy x-ray absorptiometry. The training results are shown in Table 10-1 and Figures 10-3 and 10-4. These researchers concluded that both ATM and LTM were equally effective for cardiovascular training and for producing minor reductions in body weight, as well as reductions

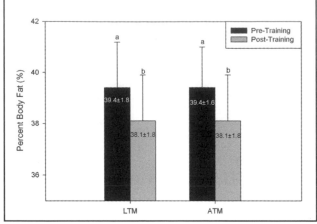

Figure 10-3. Percentage body fat before and after 12-week exercise training for both exercise training modes. Data are presented as means ±SD. Bars with different letters are significantly different (P<.05). LTM indicates land treadmill; ATM, aquatic treadmill. (Reprinted with permission from Greene NP, Lambert BS, Greene ES, Carbuhn AF, Green JS, Crouse SF. Comparative efficacy of water and land treadmill training for overweight or obese adults. *Med Sci Sports Exerc.* 2009;41:1808–1815.)

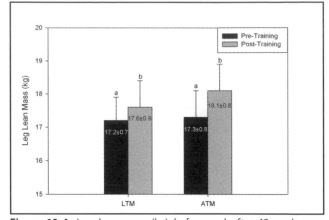

Figure 10-4. Leg lean mass (kg) before and after 12-week exercise training for both exercise training modes. Data are presented as means ±SD. Bars with different letters are significantly different (P<.05). LTM indicates land treadmill; ATM, aquatic treadmill. (Reprinted with permission from Greene NP, Lambert BS, Greene ES, Carbuhn AF, Green JS, Crouse SF. Comparative efficacy of water and land treadmill training for overweight or obese adults. *Med Sci Sports Exerc.* 2009;41:1808–1815.)

Table 10-2.

Pretraining Demographics for Subjects in the Concurrent Exercise Training Study[a]

Mode	N	Height (cm)	Weight (kg)	Age (years)	Body Mass Index	% Body Fat	VO_{2max} (mL $O_2 \cdot kg^{-1} \cdot min^{-1}$)
RT	7 (m=4 w=3)	177.9±10.9	97.3±20.3	32.4±8.7	30.4±4.6	37.8±8.3	32.5±7.8
ATM	6 (m=3 w=3)	176.5±13.9	86.9±25.3	32.7±14.3	27.3±5.0	37.1±11.4	32.4±11.2
CT	8 (m=4 w=4)	170.8±7.4	85.9±22.2	39.6±12.1	29.2±6.3	35.5±12.3	32.6±6.4
All subjects	21	174.3±10.3	90.6±21.9	35.4±11.6	29.3±5.1	35.2±10.3	32.5±8.5

[a]Values are represented as means ±SD. RT indicates resistance training group; ATM, aquatic treadmill training group; CT, concurrent resistance and aquatic treadmill training group; m, men; w, women.

in body fat (see Figure 10-3), regardless of gender. After either ATM or LTM training, VO_{2max} was significantly increased (+3.6±0.4 mLO$_2$·kg^{-1}·min^{-1}), whereas body weight (−1.2±0.3 kg), BMI (−0.56±0.11 kg·m^{-2}), percentage of body fat (−1.3%±1.3%), and fat mass (−1.1±0.3 kg) were significantly reduced. Regional leg lean body mass was significantly increased with both training modes (0.4±0.3 and 0.8±0.2 kg, respectively). Interestingly, ATM exercise but not LTM running resulted in a 0.6-kg gain in total lean body mass, a gain that nearly reached statistical significance (P=.0599). Furthermore, the leg lean mass increase was nearly twice as great after ATM training, but this difference was not significant; both exercise training modes resulted in an increase in leg lean mass (see Figure 10-4).

The results reported by Greene et al[44] that ATM exercise increased lean body mass prompted Lambert et al (S. F. Crouse, PhD, unpublished data, 2009) to study the independent and combined effects of ATM and traditional resistance training on cardiovascular, muscle strength, and body composition adaptations. Untrained men and women were recruited and tested for maximal cardiorespiratory strength and body composition variables before and after 12 weeks of training (Table 10-2). After baseline testing, each subject was randomly assigned to train in 1 of 3 groups: (1) ATM training only 3 times per week, (2) resistance training (RT) only 2 times per week, or (3) concurrent resistance (2 times per week) and ATM training (3 times per week) performed together (CT). The ACSM recommendations for exercise prescription were generally followed for ATM training frequency, intensity, and duration and also for the muscle groups, sets, repetitions, and intensity of resistance training.[2] Subjects in the CT group performed the same resistance exercise program as subjects in the RT group but additionally performed ATM exercise after each

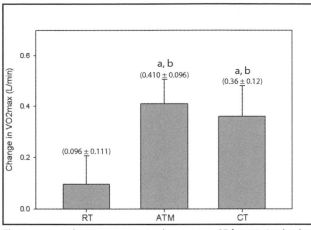

Figure 10-5. Values are represented as means ± SE for gain in absolute VO_{2max} (L/min) following 12 weeks of training. RT indicates resistance training; ATM, aquatic treadmill training; CT, concurrent RT and ATM. A indicates significantly different from pretraining; B, significantly different from the RT group. Type I error set at P < .05. (Reprinted with permission from Crouse SF.)

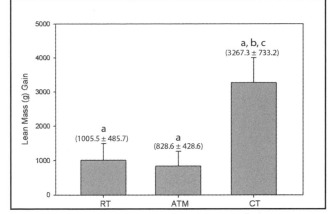

Figure 10-6. Values are represented as means ± SE for lean mass gain following 12 weeks of training. RT indicates resistance training; ATM, aquatic treadmill training; CT, concurrent RT and ATM. A indicates significantly different from baseline; B, significantly different from the RT group; C, significantly different from the ATM group. Type I error set at P < .05. (Reprinted with permission from Crouse SF.)

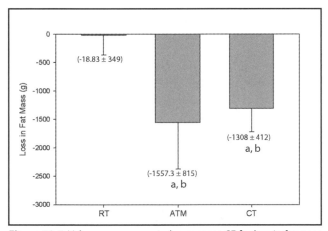

Figure 10-7. Values are represented as means ± SE for loss in fat mass following 12 weeks of training. RT indicates resistance training; ATM, aquatic treadmill training; CT, concurrent RT and ATM. A indicates significantly different from baseline; B, significantly different from the RT group. Type I error set at P < .05. (Reprinted with permission from Crouse SF.)

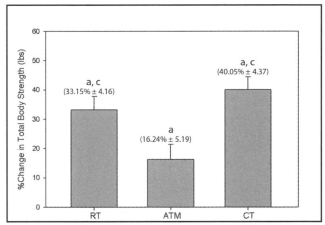

Figure 10-8. Values are represented as means ± SE for percentage gain in total body strength (calculated from the sum of 1 RM values for leg press, chest press, leg curl, lat pull, leg ext, triceps pushdown, and biceps curl) following 12 weeks of training. RT indicates resistance training; ATM, aquatic treadmill training; CT, concurrent RT and ATM. A indicates significantly different from baseline, C, significantly different from the ATM group. Type I error set at P < .05. (Reprinted with permission from Crouse SF.)

RT session until the caloric expenditure reached 500 kcal, a caloric expenditure equivalent to that expended by those in the ATM-only group. These CT subjects also completed a third training session each week in which they only performed ATM exercise. Thus, the volume of training (1500 kcal/week) was equivalent for the CT and ATM subjects, and the resistance training program was equivalent for the CT and RT subjects.

As expected, the preliminary results show that ATM and CT were the most effective means of raising VO_{2max} (Figure 10-5), because subjects in both of these exercise training groups experienced a considerably higher aerobic component in their regular training programs compared to those in the RT group. The most novel and important findings from this study were that combining RT with ATM

was the most effective means of improving lean body mass and muscle strength as well as reducing body fat (Figures 10-6 to 10-8). These data also confirm those of Greene et al[44] that ATM alone is an effective mode of exercise to reduce body fat and gain lean body mass. Indeed, the gain in lean body mass from pretraining values after ATM training alone in the CT study was only slightly, and not significantly, less than that from RT alone. It is noteworthy that these beneficial changes occurred without nutrition or diet intervention. Thus, adult men and women who wish to improve aerobic and muscular fitness should be encouraged to engage in a combination of ATM and resistance training to maximize their training benefits.

Benefits of Aquatic Treadmill Exercise in Osteoarthritis Patients

An estimated 15% of Americans have some form of arthritis, and osteoarthritis is the most common form.[46] In addition to traditional land-based exercise therapy, the use of the aquatic environment has also been advocated to facilitate exercise programming for individuals with orthopedic conditions such as osteoarthritis (OA).[47] The unique characteristics of water (hydrodynamic forces of buoyancy and added drag resistance) make it possible to potentially expend greater amounts of energy[48,49] while still reducing stress and impact forces on the lower extremity joints.[50,51]

Previous research examining the effectiveness of aquatic therapy exercise in comparison to land-based exercise in OA patients has yielded mixed results.[43,52,53] Oftentimes aquatic therapy programs are conducted in shallow or deep water pools and tend to focus on stationary arm and leg exercises to promote ROM and muscle strengthening activities with limited endurance conditioning such as water walking/jogging. An ATM has not been employed as an exercise mode and therefore water depth and gait speed have not been controlled. The mixed results reported in the literature may in part be related to this lack of control over exercise intensity. One of the challenges with prescribing underwater treadmill exercise in OA patients is determining a gait speed that may lead to therapeutic gains. Hall et al[49] reported that at treadmill speeds of 1.25 and 1.53 m/sec, VO_2 was greater in water than on land for healthy females, and when walking speeds were below 0.97 m/sec, VO_2 values were lower in water than on land in patients with rheumatoid arthritis.[36] Due to pain and other demobilizing factors of OA, it is unknown whether OA patients will be able to produce the same VO_2 response on an underwater treadmill versus a LTM matched for speed. Accordingly, it is important to standardize walking speeds between land and water to truly compare the cardiorespiratory and perceived pain responses during underwater and LTM exercise.

In view of these forgoing limitations of previous research,[54] subjects were examined to analyze the acute effects of 3 exercise sessions of ATM and LTM exercise on VO_2, perceived pain, gait kinematics during self-selected walking speed (SSP) on land, and timed up and go performance in knee OA patients. Subjects walked for 5 min each at 3 speeds: SSP, SSP + 0.13 m/sec, SSP + 0.26 m/sec. The SSPs on land were similar following the water (0.76 ± 0.24 m/sec) and land (0.80 ± 0.26 m/sec) exercise sessions.

The VO_2 values were not different between ATM exercise and LTM running at SSP + 0.26 but were significantly greater by 37% during the LTM versus ATM SSP. Perceived pain and timed up and go gain scores were 140% and 240% greater, respectively, following LTM compared to ATM exercise. Gait kinematics (ie, stride rate and stride length) were not affected by exercise conditions.

These results suggest that fluid resistance of water was not substantial enough at the slower walking speeds to counteract the cardiorespiratory relief created by the force of buoyancy. This contention is supported by previous research that indicated that buoyancy dominates at walking speeds less than 0.97 m/sec and that less energy is expended in water than on land.[36] However, when speeds are greater than 0.97 m/sec, fluid resistance may dominate and energy expenditures are similar between water and LTM exercise.[36,48,49,55]

One of the most important outcome measures in determining the efficacy of any physical therapy treatment for OA patients is reduced pain.[56,57] Denning et al[54] observed that perceived joint pain was less after aquatic versus land exercise, suggesting that underwater treadmill exercise may be efficacious for OA patients. The reduced impact forces may account for this observation. Barela and Duarte[50] reported a lower ground reaction force (GRF) and a slower stride frequency for elderly individuals while walking in water immersed to the xyphoid process compared to on land. Water depth can have a profound effect on mitigating GRFs during walking; Roesler et al[58] demonstrated a significant reduction in GRFs of 21%, 24%, and 29% for manubrium, mid-sternum, and xyphoid-level water depths compared to walking on land. If OA patients experience less pain and greater mobility after ATM walking with VO_2 values comparable to those of LTM walking, this mode of aquatic physical therapy may be suitable for treating OA patients.

Muscle Recruitment Patterns in Aquatic Treadmill Exercise Compared to Land Treadmill Exercise

Though running in ATM provides an exercise mode that appears to mimic LTM running, the combined effect of buoyancy and drag forces provides an environment where muscle recruitment patterns might be quite different. Silvers, Dickin, and Dolny (unpublished written observations, 2008) evaluated the EMG activity of selected lower extremity muscles (tibialis anterior [TA], vastus medialis [VM], rectus femoris [RF1 and RF2], biceps femoris [BF], and gastrocnemius [GAS]) during running at 3 speeds (6.5, 7.5, and 8.5 mph) in an ATM and on an LTM. EMG was expressed as a percentage of maximum voluntary contraction (%MVC) and relative to LTM activity (%LTM).

There were no significant differences in TA, BF, RF2 %MVC between LTM and ATM. There were significant differences in GAS and VM %MVC between modalities (LTM > ATM), though the initial contraction phase of RF (RF1) was greater in ATM versus LTM. The analysis of running speed indicated a significant difference in TA, BF, RF1, and RF2 %MVC for both modalities ($228.0 > 201.2 > 174.4$ m·min^{-1}) but not for GAS and VM. For both RF phases, the main effect of speed indicated significant differences across speeds ($228.0 > 201.2 > 174.4$ m·min^{-1}).

A reference activation value (percentage relative to LTM) was calculated for each muscle at all ATM running speeds. Reference activation for TA, BF, VM, and RF1 indicated a greater amount of activation during ATM exercise than LTM running at all speeds. Reference activation for all of these muscles, except the VM, tended to decrease with speed. Conversely, VM %LTM increased with speed. Reference activation for GAS and RF2 indicated a reduced amount of activation for ATM exercise compared to LTM running at all speeds. Reference activation for GAS was similar across speeds.

During ATM, RF1 activation began approximately 12% earlier in the stride cycle compared to LTM. This was in contrast with observations during DWR. Padilla et al[60] reported RF1 activity 50% later in the DWR stride cycle. However, the difference in RF1 onset was attributed to the lack of a ground support phase, which may alter lower extremity kinematics during DWR.[25]

In summary, the lower extremity muscle recruitment patterns during ATM exercise possess many characteristics of those observed for running on land. Any differences are likely a result of reduced GRFs and/or increased resistance due to drag forces.

CARDIORESPIRATORY RESPONSES TO AQUATIC TREADMILL EXERCISE BY TRAINED INDIVIDUALS

Trained Runners at Submaximal Speeds on Aquatic Treadmill

Rutledge et al[55] demonstrated that the addition of water jet resistance significantly increased the cardiorespiratory (VO$_2$ and HR) cost of ATM. While subjects ran on an ATM at speeds equal to 6.5, 7.5, and 8.5 mph, with an increase in water jet resistance from 0% to 50% and 50% to 75% ATM jet capacity, metabolic rate (VO$_2$) significantly increased on average 14.3% and 12.4%, respectively. This increase in metabolic rate is comparable to increasing running speed approximately 1.1 mph on land. Through the incorporation of water jet resistance, the ATM allows for greater metabolic stress to be placed on the individual without adding an orthopedic stress of running at a faster velocity. This allows subjects to maintain exercise intensities at a time when orthopedic conditions would normally restrict conditioning activities.

Peak Cardiorespiratory Responses in Trained Individuals to Aquatic Treadmill Exercise

One often-cited consequence of using DWR or SWR as an exercise mode is that peak or maximal HRs and oxygen consumption values are significantly lower (90% and 87%, respectively, for DWR; 84% and 94% for SWR) compared to LTM exercise.[7] Typically these conditions require subjects to perform DWR or SWR at a set leg stride cadence with increases in a step fashion until the subjects' cadence reaches a maximum. Several explanations have been proposed to explain the lower peak values in water (ie, hydrostatic effect of water, subjects determining exercise intensity, less muscle mass recruitment due to lack of ground support phase of gait). Most studies have utilized a self-selected stride rate that may erroneously assume that a maximal effort is put forth. The use of an ATM has the benefits of producing reductions in GRFs due to buoyancy and providing increased drag forces as stride characteristics that may mimic land more closely than DWR or SWR.

Silvers et al[38] evaluated the ability of an ATM to produce a cardiorespiratory challenge comparable to LTM running in recreationally active subjects. ATM increases workload presented to subjects through increasing LTM running speed and/or adding fluid resistance through the use of therapeutic jets. For this study, participants began the test, running at their predetermined initial speed, with 40% water jet resistance for 1 min. Thereafter, speed was increased 13.4 m·min^{-1} every minute for 4 min to a maximum of 206.8 ± 23.0 m·min^{-1}, with water jet resistance remaining constant at 40%. Once maximum speed was reached, water jet resistance was incrementally increased 10% every minute until volitional exhaustion. This protocol was patterned after previously established land-based treadmill protocols that initially increase running speed to a predetermined level and then increase LTM incline to fatigue. The incremental increase in treadmill speed followed by increases in water jet resistance corresponded to some degree to the increase in treadmill speed and incline experienced with typical LTM protocols.

Table 10-3 shows the peak values during LTM and ATM protocols. With the exception of expired ventilation and breath rate, the mean cardiorespiratory responses were essentially identical.

Performing exercise with ATM decreases the frontal resistance of forward locomotion (eg, participants run in place while the treadmill belt moved below) and may help to elicit a gait and muscle recruitment pattern comparable with that seen on land. Second, the ATM allowed us to administer workloads during the ATM protocol via manipulation of treadmill speed and adjustable fluid resistance (eg, water jets) as well as customize the water height to ensure that each participant was submerged to the xyphoid

Table 10-3.

Comparison of Peak Cardiorespiratory Responses During Land Treadmill and Aquatic Treadmill Protocols in Recreationally Active Subjects[a]

Variable Measured	Land Treadmill	Aquatic Treadmill	
	Mean (SD)	*Mean (SD)*	**P Value**
VO_2 ($mL \cdot kg^{-1} \cdot min^{-1}$)	52.5 (8.4)	52.8 (7.7)	.46
HR (bpm)	190.0 (11.4)	188.8 (10.4)	.30
LA (mM)	12.1 (2.5)	12.2 (2.6)	.91
V_E ($L \cdot min^{-1}$)	124.4 (29.9)	135.2 (30.0)	.00*
V_T ($L \cdot min^{-1}$)	2.48 (0.60)	2.46 (0.55)	.72
$Breaths \cdot min^{-1}$	50.0 (6.7)	55.3 (6.2)	.00*
RER	1.17 (0.05)	1.15 (0.04)	.11
RPE	18.7 (1.3)	18.4 (1.4)	.29
Test time (min)	8.7 (1.2)	8.8 (1.5)	.84
Final speed ($m \cdot min^{-1}$)	205.3 (22.3)	206.8 (23.0)	.63

[a]Values are means ± SD. VO_2 indicates oxygen uptake; HR, heart rate; LA, lactic acid; VE, minute ventilation; VT, tidal volume; RER, respiratory exchange ratio; RPE, ratings of perceived exertion; *difference between land and ATM trials were statistically different from each other.

Reprinted with permission from Silvers W, Rutledge E, Dolny D. Peak cardiorespiratory responses during aquatic and land treadmill exercise. *Med Sci Sports Exerc.* 2007;39:969–975.

level. At this water level, the forearm and a portion of the arm were submerged throughout arm swing. Moving the arms through water likely required more energy expenditure than on land. Combined with an open-ended testing timeline, we feel that the ATM afforded each participant an opportunity to exercise to his maximal potential.

These results are also highly reproducible, as demonstrated by nearly identical VO_{2peak} values (mean of 3.65 versus 3.67 $L \cdot min^{-1}$) and maximum HRs (mean of 187 versus 187 bpm) reported when 2 ATM maximal protocol tests were administered within 1 week of each other in recreationally trained subjects.[60]

ATM can elicit peak cardiorespiratory responses similar to those seen during land-based treadmill running, provided that an appropriate balance is struck between buoyancy and fluid resistance (as dictated by water submersion level and/or adjustable fluid resistance levels). Further testing with an ATM should investigate cardiorespiratory responses using different combinations of water submersion and fluid resistance during maximal exercise intensity protocols. In light of these findings, ATM training can be a viable training alternative to maintain and/or improve fitness levels for injured and healthy athletes alike.

CONCLUSION

The summary of the literature dealing with aerobic movements in water suggests that aquatic exercise has proven physical fitness and health benefits, at least in older women and some patient populations, although more research is needed in adult men. The recently developed variable-speed ATM system with adjustable water depth and frontal resistance provided by pump-driven directional water jets presents distinct advantages compared to more traditional modes of aquatic exercise. This system provides the benefit common to other aquatic exercise modes, in that water buoyancy allows for an unloading effect during walking and jogging, thus reducing joint stress and consequent joint injury, especially in the obese and those recovering from joint injury or surgery. A second and distinct benefit is that the walking or running intensity can be precisely and reproducibly controlled through operator command over the treadmill velocity and jet resistance. The ATM has proven to be a mode of exercise that can elicit a cardiorespiratory response comparable to LTM exercise. The added benefit of buoyancy and drag resistance in water has the potential to decrease joint stress and increase muscle mass in the lower extremity, respectively. Through the incorporation of water jet resistance, ATM allows for a greater metabolic stress to be placed on the individual without the additional orthopedic stress of running at a faster velocity.

Combining RT with ATM is the most effective means of improving lean body mass and muscle strength, as well as reducing body fat. These data also confirm those of Greene et al[44] that ATM alone is an effective mode of exercise to reduce body fat and gain lean body mass.

Although the published literature is sparse, it is clear that the results of ATM studies vary considerably. The variability is likely due to interstudy differences in such factors as the physical fitness status and age of the subjects; the depth of the water in the ATM; the exercise protocol, including the ambulation velocity and whether or not there are resistive jets employed in the ATM system; and the water temperature.[6] It is important that practitioners and clinicians appreciate the factors that affect physiologic responses to submaximal ATM exercise so that they may account for them in their exercise prescriptions to ensure the safety of their patients and clients. Future research should build upon the initial studies examining the effects of ATM training programs including individuals with orthopedic and metabolic diseases.

REFERENCES

1. Haskell WL, Lee IM, Pate RR, et al. Physical activity and public health: updated recommendation for adults from the American College of Sports Medicine and the American Heart Association. *Med Sci Sports Exerc.* 2007;39:1423–1434.

2. Thompson WR, Gordon NF, Pescatello LS, eds. *ACSM's Guidelines for Exercise Testing and Prescription.* Philadelphia: Lippincott Williams & Wilkins; 2010.

3. Dowzer CN, Reilly T, Cable NT. Effects of deep and shallow water running on spinal shrinkage. *Br J Sports Med.* 1998;32:44–48.

4. Frangolias DD, Rhodes EC. Metabolic responses and mechanisms during water immersion running and exercise. *Sports Med.* 1996;22:38–53.

5. Salzman A. Aquatic exercise statistics - how popular is non-swimming aquatic exercise? The Aquatic Therapist Web site. http://www.aquatictherapist.com/index/2009/04/aquatic-exercise-statistics-how-popular-is-nonswimming-aquatic-exercise.html. Published April 30, 2009. Accessed June 3, 2013.

6. Barbosa TM, Marinho DA, Reis VM, Silva AJ, Bragada JA. Physiological assessment of head-out aquatic exercises in healthy subjects: a qualitative review. *J Sports Sci Med.* 2009;8:179–189.

7. Reilly T, Dowzer C, Cable NT. The physiology of deep-water running. *J Sports Sci.* 2003;21:959–972.

8. Sheldahl LM, Tristani FE, Clifford PS, Hughes CV, Sobocinski KA, Morris RD. Effect of head-out water immersion on cardiorespiratory response to dynamic exercise. *J Am Coll Cardiol.* 1987;10:1254–1258.

9. Benelli P, Ditroilo M, De Vito G. Physiological responses to fitness activities: a comparison between land-based and water aerobics exercise. *J Strength Cond Res.* 2004;18:719–722.

10. Evans EM, Cureton KJ. Metabolic, circulatory, and perceptual responses to bench stepping in water. *J Strength Cond Res.* 1998;12:95–100.

11. Darby LA, Yaekle BC. Physiological responses during two types of exercise performed on land and in the water. *J Sports Med Phys Fitness.* 2000;40:303–311.

12. Bocalini DS, Serra AJ, Murad N, Levy RF. Water- versus land-based exercise effects on physical fitness in older women. *Geriatr Gerontol Int.* 2008;8:265–271.

13. Takeshima N, Rogers ME, Watanabe E, et al. Water-based exercise improves health-related aspects of fitness in older women. *Med Sci Sports Exerc.* 2002;33:544–551.

14. Colado JC, Triplett NT, Tella V, Saucedo P, Abellan J. Effects of aquatic resistance training on health and fitness in postmenopausal women. *Eur J Appl Physiol.* 2009;106:113–122.

15. Volaklis KA, Spassis AT, Tokmakidis SP. Land versus water exercise in patients with coronary artery disease: effects on body composition, blood lipids, and physical fitness. *Am Heart J.* 2007;154:560.e1–6.

16. Wadell K, Sundelin G, Henriksson-Larsen K, Lundgren R. High intensity physical group training in water—an effective training modality for patients with COPD. *Respir Med.* 2004;98:428–438.

17. Butts NK, Tucker M, Greening C. Physiological responses to maximal treadmill and deep water running in men and women. *Am J Sports Med.* 1991;19:612–614.

18. Butts NK, Tucker M, Smith R. Maximal responses to treadmill and deep water running in high school female cross country runners. *Res Q Exerc Sport.* 1991;62:236–239.

19. Dowzer CN, Reilly T, Cable NT, Nevill A. Maximal physiological responses to deep and shallow water running. *Ergonomics.* 1999;42:275–281.

20. Frangolias DD, Rhodes EC. Maximal and ventilatory threshold responses to treadmill and water immersion running. *Med Sci Sports Exerc.* 1995;27:1007–1013.

21. Michaud TJ, Rodriguez-Zayas J, Andres FF, Flynn MG, Lambert CP. Comparative exercise responses of deep-water and treadmill running. *J Strength Cond Res.* 1995;9:104–109.

22. Nakanishi Y, Kimura T, Yokoo Y. Maximal physiological responses to deep water running at thermoneutral temperature. *Appl Human Sci.* 1999;18:31–35.

23. Svedenhag J, Seger J. Running on land and in water: comparative exercise physiology. *Med Sci Sports Exer.* 1992;24:1155–1160.

24. Town GP, Bradley SS. Maximal metabolic responses of deep and shallow-water running in trained runners. *Med Sci Sports Exerc.* 1991;23:238–241.

25. Killgore GL, Wilcox AR, Caster BL, Wood TM. A lower-extremities kinematic comparison of deep-water running styles and treadmill running. *J Strength Cond Res.* 2006;20:919–927.

26. Kilding AE, Scott MA, Mullineaux DR. A kinematic comparison of deep water running and overground running in endurance runners. *J Strength Cond Res.* 2007;21:476–480.

27. Reilly T, Cable NT, Dowzer CN. The effects of a 6 week land- and water-running training programme on aerobic, anaerobic and muscle strength measures. *J Sports Sci.* 2003;21:333–334.

28. Meredith-Jones K, Legge M, Jones LM. Circuit based deep water running improves cardiovascular fitness, strength and abdominal obesity in older, overweight women. *Med Sport.* 2009;13:5–12.

29. Broman G, Quintana M, Lindberg T, Jansson E, Kaijser L. High intensity deep water training can improve aerobic power in elderly women. *Eur J Appl Physiol.* 2006;98:117–123.

30. Assis MR, Silva LE, Alves AMB, et al. A randomized controlled trial of deep water running: clinical effectiveness of aquatic exercise to treat fibromyalgia. *Arthritis Rheum.* 2006;55:57–65.

31. Kaneda K, Wakabayashi H, Sato D, Nomura T. Lower extremity muscle activity during different types and speeds of underwater movement. *J Physiol Anthropol.* 2007;26:197–200.

32. Kaneda K, Wakabayashi H, Sato D, Uekusa T, Nomura T. Lower extremity muscle activity during deep-water running on self-determined pace. *J Electromyogr Kinesiol.* 2008;18:965–972.

33. Kaneda K, Sato D, Wakabayashi H, Nomura T. EMG activity of hip and trunk muscles during deep-water running. *J Electromyogr Kinesiol.* 2009;19:1064–1070.

34. Greene NP, Greene ES, Carbuhn AF, Green JS, Crouse SF. VO2 prediction and cardiorespiratory responses during underwater treadmill exercise. *Res Q Exerc Sport.* 2011;82(2):264–273.

35. Fujishima K, Shimizu T. Body temperature, oxygen uptake and heart rate during walking in water and on land at an exercise intensity based on RPE in elderly men. *J Physiol Anthropol.* 2003;22:83–88.

36. Hall J, Grant J, Blake D, Taylor G, Garbutt G. Cardiorespiratory responses to aquatic treadmill walking in patients with rheumatoid arthritis. *Physiother Res Int.* 2004;9:59–73.

37. Dolbow DR, Farley RS, Kim JK, Caputo JL. Oxygen consumption, heart rate, rating of perceived exertion, and systolic blood pressure with water treadmill walking. *J Aging Phys Act.* 2008;16:14–23.

38. Silvers W, Rutledge E, Dolny D. Peak cardiorespiratory responses during aquatic and land treadmill exercise. *Med Sci Sports Exerc.* 2007;39:969–975.

39. Hall C, Figueroa A, Fernhall B, Kanaley JA. Energy expenditure of walking and running: comparison with prediction equations. *Med Sci Sports Exerc.* 2004;36:2128–2134.

40. Belisle M, Roskies E, Levesque JM. Improving adherence to physical-activity. *Health Psychol.* 1987;6:159–172.

41. Blair SN, Kohl HW, Goodyear NN. Rates and risks for running and exercise injuries—studies in 3 populations. *Res Q Exerc Sport.* 1987;58:221–228.

42. Jadelis K, Miller ME, Ettinger WH, Messier SP. Strength, balance, and the modifying effects of obesity and knee pain: results from the Observational Arthritis Study in Seniors (OASIS). *J Am Geriatr Soc.* 2001;49:884–891.

43. Wang TJ, Belza B, Thompson FE, Whitney JD, Bennett K. Effects of aquatic exercise on flexibility, strength and aerobic fitness in adults with osteoarthritis of the hip or knee. *J Adv Nurs.* 2007;57:141–152.

44. Greene NP, Lambert BS, Greene ES, Carbuhn AF, Green JS, Crouse SF. Comparative efficacy of water and land treadmill training for overweight or obese adults. *Med Sci Sports Exerc.* 2009;41:1808–1815.

45. Bruce RA, Kusumi F, Hosmer D. Maximal oxygen intake and nomographic assessment of functional aerobic impairment in cardiovascular disease. *Am Heart J.* 1973;85:546–562.

46. Lawrence RC, Felson DT, Helmick CG, et al. Estimates of the prevalence of arthritis and other rheumatic conditions in the United States. Part II. *Arthritis Rheum.* 2008;58:26–35.

47. Cadmus L, Patrick MB, Maciejewski ML, Topolski T, Belza B, Patrick DL. Community-based aquatic exercise and quality of life in persons with osteoarthritis. *Med Sci Sports Exerc.* 2010;42:8–15.

48. Gleim GW, Nicholas JA. Metabolic costs and heart rate responses to treadmill walking in water at different depths and temperatures. *Am J Sports Med.* 1989;17:248–252.

49. Hall J, Macdonald IA, Maddison PJ, O'Hare JP. Cardiorespiratory responses to underwater treadmill walking in healthy females. *Eur J Appl Physiol Occup Physiol.* 1998;77:278–284.

50. Barela AM, Duarte M. Biomechanical characteristics of elderly individuals walking on land and in water. *J Electromyogr Kinesiol.* 2008;18:446–454.

51. Barela AM, Stolf SF, Duarte M. Biomechanical characteristics of adults walking in shallow water and on land. *J Electromyogr Kinesiol.* 2006;16:250–256.

52. Hinman RS, Heywood SE, Day AR. Aquatic physical therapy for hip and knee osteoarthritis: results of a single-blind randomized controlled trial. *Phys Ther.* 2007;87:32–43.

53. Lund H, Weile U, Christensen R, et al. A randomized controlled trial of aquatic and land-based exercise in patients with knee osteoarthritis. *J Rehabil Med.* 2008;40:137–144.

54. Denning W, Bressel E, Dolny D. Underwater treadmill exercise as a potential treatment for adults with osteoarthritis. *Int J Aquat Res Educ.* 2010;4:70–80.

55. Rutledge E, Silvers WM, Browder K, Dolny D. Metabolic-cost comparison of submaximal land and aquatic exercise. *Int J Aquat Res Educ.* 2007;1:118–133.

56. Edmonds S. Therapeutic targets for osteoarthritis. *Maturitas.* 2009;63:191–194.

57. Hurley MV. Muscle dysfunction and effective rehabilitation of knee osteoarthritis: what we know and what we need to find out. *Arthritis Rheum.* 2003;49:444–452.

58. Roesler H, Haupenthal A, Schutz GR, de Sousa PV. Dynamometric analysis of the maximum force applied in aquatic human gait at 1.3 m of immersion. *Gait Posture.* 2006;24:412–417.

59. Padilla JN, Mercer JA, Hreljac A, Osternig LR. Lower extremity EMG for an experienced runner during deep water running. *Med Sci Sports Exerc.* 2001;33(suppl):S315.

60. Silvers WM, Dolny DG. Reliability of peak cardiorespiratory responses during aquatic treadmill exercise. *Int J Aquat Res Exerc.* 2008;2:140–150.

Appendices

APPENDIX A

Accelerated Rehabilitation Following ACL-PTG Reconstruction

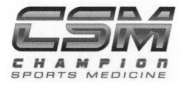

Preoperative Phase

Goals:

- Diminish inflammation, swelling, and pain
- Restore normal range of motion (especially knee extension)
- Restore voluntary muscle activation
- Protect the knee from further injury—especially menisci
- Provide patient education to prepare patient for surgery

Brace—Elastic wrap or knee sleeve to reduce swelling

Weight Bearing—As tolerated with or without crutches

Exercises:

- Ankle pumps
- Passive knee extension to zero
- Passive knee flexion to tolerance
- Straight leg raises (3 way, flexion, abduction, adduction)
- Quadriceps setting
- Closed kinetic chain exercises: mini squats, lunges, step-ups

Muscle stimulation—Electrical muscle stimulation to quadriceps during voluntary quadriceps exercises (4 to 6 hours per day)

Neuromuscular/Proprioception Training:

- Eliminate quad avoidance gait
- Retro stepping drills
- Balance training drills

Wilk KE, Joyner DM. *The Use of Aquatics in Orthopedic and Sports Medicine Rehabilitation and Physical Conditioning (pp 131-139).*
© 2014 SLACK Incorporated.

Cryotherapy/Elevation—Apply ice 20 minutes of every hour, elevate leg with knee in full extension (knee must be above heart)

Patient Education:
- Review postoperative rehabilitation program
- Review instructional video (optional)
- Select appropriate surgical date

Immediate Postoperative Phase (Day 1 to Day 7)

Goals:
- Restore full passive knee extension
- Diminish joint swelling and pain
- Restore patellar mobility
- Gradually improve knee flexion
- Re-establish quadriceps control
- Restore independent ambulation

Postoperative Day 1

Brace—Brace/immobilizer applied to knee, locked in full extension during ambulation and sleeping; unlock brace while sitting, etc.

Weight Bearing—Two crutches, weight bearing as tolerated

Exercises:
- Ankle pumps
- Overpressure into full, passive knee extension
- Active and passive knee flexion (90 degree by day 5)
- Straight leg raises (flexion, abduction, adduction)
- Quadriceps isometric setting
- Hamstring stretches
- Closed kinetic chain exercises: mini squats, weight shifts

Muscle Stimulation—Use muscle stimulation during active muscle exercises (4 to 6 hours per day)

Continuous Passive Motion—As needed, 0 to 45/50 degrees (as tolerated and as directed by physician)

Ice and Evaluation—Ice 20 minutes out of every our and elevate with knee in full extension

Postoperative Day 2 to 3

Brace—Brace/immobilizer, locked at zero degrees extension for ambulation and unlocked for sitting, etc.

Weight Bearing—Two crutches, weight bearing as tolerated

Range of Motion—Remove brace, perform range of motion exercises 4 to 6 times per day

Exercises:
- Multi-angle isometrics at 90 and 60 degrees (knee extension)
- Knee extension 90 to 40 degrees
- Overpressure into extension (knee extension should be at least 0 degrees to slight hyperextension)
- Patellar mobilization
- Ankle pumps
- Straight leg raises (3 directions)
- Mini squats and weight shifts
- Quadriceps isometric setting

Muscle Stimulation—Electrical muscle stimulation to quads (6 hours per day)

Continuous Passive Motion—0 to 90 degrees, as needed

Ice and Evaluation—Ice 20 minutes out of every hour and elevate leg with knee in full extension

Postoperative Day 4 to 7

Brace—Brace/immobilizer, locked at zero degrees extension for ambulation and unlocked for sitting, etc.

Weight Bearing—Two crutches, weight bearing as tolerated

Range of Motion—Remove brace to perform range of motion exercises 4 to 6 times per day, knee flexion 90 degrees by Day 5, approximately 100 degrees by Day 7

Exercises:
- Multi-angle isometrics at 90 and 60 degrees (knee extension)
- Knee extension 90 to 40 degrees
- Overpressure into extension (full extension 0 degrees to 5 to 7 hyperextension)
- Patellar mobilization (5 to 8 times daily)
- Ankle pumps
- Straight leg raises (3 directions)
- Mini squats and weight shifts
- Standing hamstring curls
- Quadriceps isometric setting
- Proprioception and balance activities

Neuromuscular training/proprioception—OKC passive/active joint repositioning at 90, 60 degrees; CKC squats/weight shifts with repositioning

Muscle Stimulation—Electrical muscle stimulation (continue 6 hours daily)

Continue Passive Motion—0 to 90 degrees, as needed

Ice and Elevation—Ice 20 minutes of every hour and elevate leg with knee full extension

II. Early Rehabilitation Phase (Week 2 to 4)

Criteria to Progress to Phase II
1. Quad control (ability to perform good quad set and SLR)

2. Full passive knee extension

3. PROM 0 to 90 degrees

4. Good patellar mobility

5. Minimal joint effusion

6. Independent ambulation

Goals:

- Maintain full passive knee extension (at least 0 to 5 to 7 hyperextension)
- Gradually increase knee flexion
- Diminish swelling and pain
- Muscle control and activation
- Restore proprioception/neuromuscular control
- Normalize patellar mobility

Week 2

Brace—Continue locked brace for ambulation and sleeping

Weight Bearing—As tolerated (goal is to discontinue crutches 10 to 14 days post op)

Passive Range of Motion—Self-range of motion (ROM) stretching (4 to 5 times daily), emphasis on maintaining full, passive ROM
*Restore patient's symmetrical extension

KT 2000 Test (15 lb. anterior-posterior test only)

Exercises:

- Muscle stimulation to quadriceps exercises
- Isometric quadriceps sets
- Straight leg raises (4 planes)
- Leg press (0 to 60 degrees)
- Knee extension 90 to 40 degrees
- Half squats (0 to 40)
- Weight shifts
- Front and side lunges
- Hamstring curls standing (active ROM)
- Bicycle (if ROM allows)
- Proprioception training
- Overpressure into extension
- Passive ROM from 0 to 100 degrees
- Patellar mobilization
- Well leg exercises
- Progressive resistance extension program—start with 1 lb, progress 1 lb per week

Proprioception/Neuromuscular Training
- OKC passive/active joint repositioning 90, 60, 30 degrees
- CKC joint repositioning during squats/lunges
- Initiate squats on tilt board

Swelling control—Ice, compression, elevation

Pool Exercises—(use protective cover over incision if needed) walking in water up to axilla, minisquats, weight shifts, lateral movements, knee flexion, knee extension, and hip abd/adduction and extension

Week 3

Brace—Discontinue locked brace (some patients use ROM brace for ambulation). If patient continues to use brace, unlock brace for ambulation

Passive ROM—Continue ROM stretching and overpressure into extension (ROM should be 0 to 100/105 degrees)
*Restore patients symmetrical extension

Exercises:
- Continue all exercises as in Week 2
- Passive ROM 0 to 105 degrees
- Bicycle for range of motion stimulus and endurance
- Pool walking program (if incision is closed)
- Eccentric quadriceps program 40 to 100 (isotonic only)
- Lateral lunges (straight plane)
- Front step downs
- Lateral step-overs (cones)
- Stair-stepper machine
- Progress proprioception drills, neuromuscular control drills
- Continue passive/active reposition drills (CKC, OKC)

Pool Exercises: Continue above pool exercises, initiate fast pace walking, emphasize hip, hamstrings, and balance exercises

III. Progressive Strengthening/Neuromuscular Control Phase (Week 4 to 10)

Criteria to Enter Phase III:
1. Active ROM 0 to 115 degrees
2. Quadriceps strength 60% > contralateral side (isometric test at 60 degree knee flexion)
3. Unchanged KT test bilateral values (+1 or less)
4. Minimal to no full joint effusion
5. No joint line or patellofemoral pain

Goals:
- Restore full knee ROM (5 to 0 to 125 degrees) symmetrical motion
- Improve lower extremity strength
- Enhance proprioception, balance, and neuromuscular control
- Improve muscular endurance
- Restore limb confidence and function

Brace—No immobilizer or brace, may use knee sleeve to control swelling/support

ROM—Self-ROM (4 to 5 times daily using the other leg to provide ROM), emphasis on maintaining zero degrees passive extension
- PROM 0 to 125 degrees at 4 weeks

KT 2000 Test—(Week 4, 20 lb. anterior and posterior test)

Week 4

Exercises:
- Progress isometric strengthening program
- Leg Press (0 to 100 degrees)
- Knee extension 90 to 40 degrees
- Hamstring curls (isotonics)
- Hip abduction and adduction
- Hip flexion and extension
- Lateral step-overs
- Lateral lunges (straight plane and multi-plane drills)
- Lateral step ups
- Front step downs
- Wall squats
- Vertical squats
- Standing toe calf raises
- Seated toe calf raises
- Biodex stability system (balance, squats, etc)
- Proprioception drills
- Bicycle
- Stair stepper machine
- Pool program (backward running, hip and leg exercises)

Proprioception/Neuromuscular Drills
- Tilt board squats (perturbation)
- Passive/active reposition OKC
- CKC repositioning on tilt board

Pool Exercises: Continue all above pool exercises, add resistive paddles, etc.

Week 6

KT 2000 Test—20 and 30 lb anterior and posterior test

Exercises:
- Continue all exercises
- Pool running (forward) and agility drills
- Balance on tilt boards
- Progress to balance and ball throws
- Wall slides/squats

Pool Exercises: Continue all hip, hamstrings, and quadriceps exercises
Initiate forward and backward running in water depth to axilla (50% to 60% effort)

Week 8

KT 2000 Test—20 and 30 lb anterior and posterior test

Exercises:

- Continue all exercises listed in Weeks 4 to 6
- Leg press sets (single leg) 0 to 100 degrees and 40 to 100 degrees
- Plyometric leg press
- Perturbation training
- Isokinetic exercises (90 to 40 degrees) (120 to 240 degrees/second)
- Walking program
- Bicycle for endurance
- Stair stepper machine for endurance
- Biodex stability system
- Training on tilt board

Pool Exercises: Continue all hip, hamstrings, and quadriceps exercises; initiate forward and backward running in water depth to axilla (65% to 75% effort); may initiate lateral slides, carcaricos, etc.

Week 10

KT 2000 Test—20 and 30 lb and manual maximum test

Isokinetic Test—concentric knee extension/flexion at 180 and 300 degrees/second

Exercises:

- Continue all exercises listed in Weeks 6, 8, and 10
- Plyometric training drills
- Continue stretching drills
- Progress strengthening exercises and neuromuscular training

IV. Advanced Activity Phase (Week 10 to 16)

Criteria to enter Phase IV:

1. AROM 0 to 125 degrees or greater
2. Quad strength 75% of contralateral side, knee extension flexor: extensor ratio 70% to 75%
3. No change in KT values (comparable with contralateral side, within 2 mm)
4. No pain or effusion
5. Satisfactory clinical exam
6. Satisfactory isokinetic test (values at 180 degrees)
   - Quadriceps bilateral comparison 75%
   - Hamstrings equal bilateral
   - Quadriceps peak torque/body weight 65% at 180 degrees/second (males) 55% at 180 degrees/second (females)
   - Hamstrings/quadriceps ratio 66% to 75%

7. Hop test (80% of contralateral leg)

8. Subjective knee scoring (modified Noyes System) 80 points or better

Goals:

- Normalize lower extremity strength
- Enhance muscular power and endurance
- Improve neuromuscular control
- Perform selected sport-specific drills

Exercises:

- May initiate running program (weeks 10 to 12) (Physician decision)
- May initiate light sport program (golf) (Physician decision)
- Continue all strengthening drills
    - Leg press
    - Wall squats
    - Hip abd/adduction
    - Hip flex/ext
    - Knee extension 90 to 40
    - Hamstring curls
    - Standing toe calf
    - Seated toe calf
    - Step down
    - Lateral step ups
    - Lateral lunges
- Neuromuscular training
    - Lateral step-overs cones
    - Lateral lunges
    - Tilt board drills
    - Sports RAC repositioning on tilt board

Week 14 to 16

- Progress program
- Continue all drills above
- May initiate lateral agility drills
- Backward running

Pool Exercises: Continue all hip, hamstrings, and quadriceps exercises; Initiate forward and backward running in water depth to waist (90% to 100% effort); Utilize resistance of water jets, kick paddle, etc.

V. Return to Activity Phase (Month 16 to 22)

Criteria to enter Phase V:

1. Full ROM

2. Unchanged KT 2000 test (within 2.5 mm of opposite side)

3. Isokinetic test that fulfills criteria

4. Quadriceps bilateral comparison (80% or greater)

5. Hamstring bilateral comparison (110% or greater)

6. Quadriceps torque/body weight ratio (55% or greater)

7. Hamstrings/quadriceps ratio (70% or greater)

8. Proprioceptive test (100% of contralateral leg)

9. Functional test (85% or greater of contralateral side)

10. Satisfactory clinical exam

11. Subjective knee scoring (modified Noyes System) (90 points or better)

Goals:
- Gradual return to full-unrestricted sports
- Achieve maximal strength and endurance
- Normalize neuromuscular control
- Progress skill training

Tests—KT 2000, isokinetic, and functional tests before return

Exercises:
- Continue strengthening exercises
- Continue neuromuscular control drills
- Continue plyometrics drills
- Progress running and agility program
- Progress sport specific training
  - Running/cutting/agility drills
  - Gradual return to sport drills

6 Month Follow-Up	12 Month Follow-Up
Isokinetic test	Isokinetic test
KT 2000 test	KT 2000 test
Functional test	Functional test

JRA/WJC/KEW: 4/93, Revised: 5/95, 7/98, 1/01, 3/05, 9/07, 9/09, 4/11, 7/11(P).

APPENDIX B

Microfracture Procedure (Femoral Condyle)

Regular (Medium-Large Lesion) Rehabilitation Program

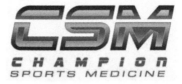

Precautions: Control weight bearing, non weight bearing forces for several weeks
   Control axial loading and shear forces
   No deep squatting, stairs with WB, and twisting

Phase I: Protection Phase

Goals:
- Reduce swelling and inflammation
- Protect and promote healing articular cartilage
- Restoration of full passive knee extension
- Gradual restoration of knee flexion
- Re-establish voluntary quadriceps control

A. Weeks 0 to 2

Brace—Use elastic wrap to control swelling and inflammation

Weight Bearing—Non weight bearing week 0 to 2
   Use of crutches to control weight bearing forces

Inflammation Control—Use of ice and compression 15 to 20 min (6 to 8 times daily)

Range of Motion (ROM):
- Immediate motion
- Full passive knee extension
- Passive and active assisted knee flexion (3 to 5 times daily) to promote articular cartilage healing
  - Week 1: 0 to 90 degrees or beyond (to tolerance)
  - Week 2: 0 to 105 degrees or beyond (to tolerance)
- Flexibility exercises: stretch hamstrings, calf, and quads

Wilk KE, Joyner DM. *The Use of Aquatics in Orthopedic and Sports Medicine Rehabilitation and Physical Conditioning (pp 141-144).*
© 2014 SLACK Incorporated.

Strengthening Exercises:

- Isometric quadriceps setting
- Straight leg raises (4 directions)
- Multi-angle quadriceps
- Electrical muscle stimulation to quads
- Bicycle when ROM permits
- Proprioception and balance training

Functional Activities—Gradual return to daily activities
Monitor swelling, pain, and loss of motion

B. Weeks 3 to 4

Weight Bearing:

- Toe-touch WB week 3
- 25% WB week 4
- Weight bearing crutches

ROM:

- Gradually progress knee flexion
  - Week 3: 0 to 115/125 degrees
  - Week 4: 0 to 125/130+ degrees
- Maintain full passive knee extension
- Continue stretches for quadriceps, hamstrings, gastroc
- Perform active assisted and active ROM (4 to 5 times daily)

Strengthening Exercises:

- Bicycles (1 to 2 times daily)
  - Low intensity bicycle = longer duration
- Quads setting
- Straight leg flexion
- Hip abd/adduction
- Hip flexion/extension
- Light hamstring curls
- Pool program (once incisions are closed)
- Proprioception and balance training
- No OKC resisted knee extension

Pool Exercises: (use protective cover over incision if needed) walking in water up to axilla, minisquats, weight shifts, lateral movements, knee flexion, knee extension, and hip abd/adduction and extension

Inflammation Control: Continue use of ice, elevation and compression (4 to 5 times daily)

Functional Activities:—Gradually return to functional activities
No sports or impact loading

Phase II: Intermediate Phase (Weeks 5 to 8)

Goals:
- Protect and promote articular cartilage healing
- Gradually increase joint stresses and loading
- Improve lower extremity strength and endurance
- Gradually increase functional activities

Weight Bearing:
- 50% WB week 6
- 75% WB week 7
- FWB as tolerated week 8

Flexibility Exercises—Continue stretching hamstrings, quadriceps, and calf

Strengthening Exercises:
- Initiate functional rehab exercises
- Minisquats and leg press Week 6
- Closed kinetic chain exercises (step-ups, lunges)

Pool Exercises: Continue all above pool exercises, add resistive paddles, etc.

Week 8

- Vertical squats, wall squats, leg press
- Bicycle, elliptical (low intensity, long duration)
- Initiate progressive resistance exercise* (PREs)
- Hip abd/adduction, extension/flexion
- Hamstring strengthening (light)
- Pool program – continue walking program, bicycling motions, hip strengthening, minisquats, calf raises
- Initiate walking program* (light walking)
- Proprioception and balance training

Functional Activities—Gradually increase walking program

   *Progression based on monitoring patient swelling, pain, and motion

Phase III: Light Activity Phase (Weeks 8 to 16)

Goals:
- Improve muscular strength/endurance
- Increase functional activities
- Gradually increase loads applied to joint
- Control compression and shear forces

Criteria to progress to phase II:
1. Full, non-painful ROM

2. Strength within 20% contralateral limb

3. Able to walk 1.5 miles or bike for 20 to 25 minutes without symptoms

Exercises:

- Continue progressive resistance exercises
- Continue functional rehabilitation exercises
- Balance and proprioception drills
- Bicycle and elliptical
- Neuromuscular control drills
- Initiate light running program (**Physician will determine)
- Continue all stretches to lower extremity

Functional Activities—Gradually increase walking distance/endurance
                        Pool running Week 10

Pool Exercises: Continue all hip, hamstrings, and quadriceps exercises
                Initiate forward and backward running in water depth to chest (60% to 75% effort)
                Utilize resistance of water jets, kick paddle, etc.

- Light running week 12 to 16
- Progress running program week 16 to 18
- Progression based on monitoring patient's swelling, pain, and motion*

Phase IV: Return to Activity Phase (Weeks 16 to 26)

Goals—Gradual return to full unrestricted functional activities
        *Actual timeframes may vary based on extent of injury and surgery
        *Physician will advise rate of progression

Exercises:

- Continue functional rehab exercises
- Continue flexibility exercises
- Restrict with deep squatting with resistance and heavy knee extensions
- Monitor jumping activities closely

Pool Exercises: Continue all hip, hamstrings, and quadriceps exercises
                Initiate forward and backward running in water depth to waist (90% to 100% effort)
                Utilize resistance of water jets, kick paddle, etc.

Functional Activities:

- Low impact sports (cycling, golf) weeks 6 to 8
- Moderate impact sports (jogging, tennis, aerobics) weeks 12 to 16
- High impact sports (basketball, soccer, volleyball) weeks 16 to 26
    * Actual return to sports or strenuous will be determined by your Physician and rehabilitation team

JRA/KEW: 4/04, Revised: 7/08, 1/09, 4/11, 7/11 (P)

APPENDIX C

Total Hip Replacement: Aquatic Therapy Protocol

The following is to be used as a guideline in progressing patient's status post total hip reconstruction. Each patient's specific needs, response to treatment, and comorbidities should be assessed determining the specific course of treatment. Refer to Total Hip Protocol for specific precautions.

Initial visit through the end of the first week:

- Appropriate bio-occlusive dressing is applied.
- Primary focus in first week of treatment is to control swelling, decrease pain, and introduce motion.
- Initiate gentle lower extremity range of motion (ROM). Patient is encouraged not to force motion, but rather to gently move through a comfortable ROM. Reinforce Total Hip Precautions through our treatment.
  - Seated knee flexion and ankle pumps
  - Heel/toe lifts
  - Gentle mini squats, not past 70 degrees of hip flexion
  - Gentle and slow hip abduction, ensure that patient does not return to full adduction
  - Gentle hip circles
- Begin gentle ambulation (suggest .5 mph x 5 min).

Second through end of third week:

- Continue with above exercises.
- D/C bio-occlusive dressing when all steri-strips have fallen off or have been taken off and wound is well healed.
- Focus on gentle strengthening and ROM exercises:
  - Standing hip flexion and extension
  - Marching in place
  - Hamstring stretch
  - Calf stretch
  - Step ups/downs side/side from platform to deeper water
- Increase ambulation speed and time by approximately 2 mph and by 2 min per day, add jets for resistance as patient tolerates.

Fourth through sixth weeks:

- Continue with above exercises.
- Add swim fins, aqua socks, or balance rings for resistance.
- Alternating lunges not past 70 degrees of hip flexion.
- Upper extremity resistance for challenges to balance and core stabilization.

Wilk KE, Joyner DM. *The Use of Aquatics in Orthopedic and Sports Medicine Rehabilitation and Physical Conditioning (pp 145-146).*
© 2014 SLACK Incorporated.

- Hip hikes from step to strength hip stabilizers.
- Patient to begin walking step over, step up, and down pool stairs.
- Massage jets to decrease swelling, decrease muscle spasms, and scar massage.

Appendix D

Total Knee Replacement: Aquatic Therapy Protocol

The following is to be used as guideline in progressing patient's status post total knee reconstruction. Each patient's specific needs, response to treatment, and comorbidities should be assessed in determining the specific course of treatment.

Initial visit:

- Appropriate bio-occlusive dressing is applied.
- Initiate gentle knee flexion. Patient is encouraged not to try to force the motion initially, but rather to gently move through a comfortable range of motion (ROM) and slowly build on that motion as pain allows.
  - Mini squats
  - Seated alternating gentle kicks
  - Long arc quads from sitting position on step
  - Gentle lunge with operative leg on step
- Begin gentle ambulation (suggest .5 mph x 5 min).
- Focus on hamstring stretch and gastroc/soleus stretches.

Second visit through third week:

- Continue with above exercises.
- D/C bio-occlusive dressing when all steri-strips have fallen off or been taken off and wound is well healed.
- Initiate hip ROM and strengthening with hip flexion and extension, ab/adduction
- Initiate joint mobilization in pool.
- Increase ambulation speed and time by approximately 2 mph and 2 minutes per day until up to 2 mph and 10 minutes. Use caution increasing speed above 2 mph due to decreased quad strength making is difficult for the operative knee to keep that pace with good mechanics and the resistance of the water.
- To increase effort of ambulation, increase jets. Be sure resistance is aimed at the patient's trunk or chest, not below the knee.

Fourth through sixth weeks:

- Continue with above exercises.
- Add swim fins, aqua socks, or balance rings for resistance.
- Alternating lunges.
- Patient to begin walking up and down pool stairs, step over step.
- Balance activities (ie, single leg stance, tandem stance).
- Upper extremity resistance for postural control and strengthening.
- Massage jets to decrease swelling, relax soft tissue, and to perform scar massage.

Wilk KE, Joyner DM. *The Use of Aquatics in Orthopedic and Sports Medicine Rehabilitation and Physical Conditioning (p 147).*

Appendix E

Nonoperative Treatment of Osteoarthritis of the Knee

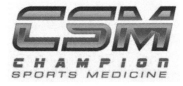

The Rehabilitation Program

The Acute Phase

Goals:
- Decrease pain and inflammation
- Improve range of motion (ROM) and flexibility
- Enhance lower extremity muscular strength
- Modification of activities
- Alter applied joint forces

Decrease pain and inflammation
- NSAIDs
- ROM exercises
- Cryotherapy

Improve ROM and flexibility
- Restore full passive knee extension
  - Overpressure into extension
  - Hamstring stretches
  - Gastrocnemius stretches
- Gradually increase knee flexion
  - AAROM knee flexion
  - Quadriceps stretches
  - PROM flexion

Wilk KE, Joyner DM. *The Use of Aquatics in Orthopedic and Sports Medicine Rehabilitation and Physical Conditioning (pp 149-152).* © 2014 SLACK Incorporated.

Enhance lower extremity muscular strength

- Quads, hamstrings, hip, and calf
- Gradual program (moderate intensity exercise)
  - Quad sets
  - SLR flexion (use ankle weights when able)
  - Initiate leg extensions 0 to 90 degrees (if painful, implement patellar protection program)
  - Hip abd/adduction
  - Knee extension
  - ¼ squats
  - Bicycle (high seat and easy resistance) long duration cycling
- Pool Program: walking program in water depth to chest; lower extremity exercises: quadriceps, hip abd/adduction, extension, mini squats, weight shifts, single-leg cycling motion, arm circles, diagonal patterns, etc.

Modification of activities

- No excessive joint compression forces
- No excessive joint shear forces
- No repetitive pounding activities (running)
- Use of pool for exercise

Alter applied joint forces

- Assess varus deformity
  - Lateral heel wedges
  - Osteoarthritis knee braces
  - Shoe insoles to control ground reaction forces
  - Shoe modifications: walking shoe—jogging shoe

Nutritional supplements

- Proper nutrition
- Multivitamin
- Increase water consumption
- Supplements
- Glucosamine with chondroitin sulfate (may be beneficial)

The Subacute Phase

Goals:

- Improve ROM and flexibility
- Enhance lower extremity muscular strength
- Improve muscular endurance
- Gradual return to functional activities

Improve flexibility

- Continue stretching exercises
  - Hamstrings
  - Hip flexors, IT band
  - Quadriceps
  - Calf

Enhance muscular strength
- Gradually increase program
  - Quad sets
  - ¼ squats
  - Wall squats
  - Front lunges
  - Lateral steps-ups (low step)
  - Bicycle (gradually increase time)
- Enhance endurance
  - Bicycle (longer duration)
  - Increase repetitions
  - Pool program

- Pool Program: gradually increase walking program (decrease depth of water to waist or slightly above and increase intensity 65% to 75%), continue lower extremity exercises, initiate resistance through kick boards, paddles, and ankle paddles. May begin swimming program and upper extremity exercises.

- Gradual return to functional activities
  - Walking program
  - No running
  - Golf, tennis

The Chronic Phase

Goals:
- Maintain/improve flexibility
- Gradually improve muscular strength
- Gradually return to functional activities

Flexibility exercises:
- Continue stretches before/after exercise program
- Improve muscular strength
- Strengthening program without symptoms
  - Quad sets
  - ½ squats
  - Wall squats
  - Lunges
  - Bicycles

- Pool Program: gradually increase walking program (decrease depth of water to waist or slightly above, and increase intensity 75% to 80%).
  Perform forward/backward walking, lateral movements, etc.
  Progress lower extremity exercises, initiate resistance through kick boards, paddles, and ankle paddles. May begin swimming program and upper extremity exercises.

Functional activities

- Continue activities which are pain-free and asymptomatic
- Watch for swelling, morning stiffness
- Continue exercise program 3 to 4 times per week

KEW, JRA: 6/10, 7/11(P)

APPENDIX F

Arthroscopic Anterior Bankart Repair

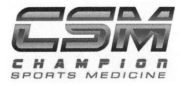

I. Phase I: Immediate Postoperative Phase "Restrictive Motion" (Weeks 0 to 6)

Goals:
- Protect the anatomic repair
- Prevent negative effects of immobilization
- Promote dynamic stability and proprioception
- Diminish pain and inflammation

Weeks 0 to 2

- Sling for 4 weeks
- Sleep in immobilizer for 4 weeks
- Elbow/hand range of motion (ROM)
- Hand gripping exercises
- Passive and gentle active assistive ROM exercise
  - Flexion to 70 degrees week 1
  - Flexion to 90 degrees week 2
  - ER/IR with arm 30 degrees abduction
    - ER to 5 to 10 degrees
    - IR to 45 degrees
    - **NO active ER or Extension or Abduction
- Submaximal isometrics for shoulder musculature (on land and in pool)
- Rhythmic stabilization drills ER/IR
- Proprioception drills
- Cryotherapy, modalities as indicated

Wilk KE, Joyner DM. *The Use of Aquatics in Orthopedic
and Sports Medicine Rehabilitation and Physical Conditioning (pp 153-156).*
© 2014 SLACK Incorporated.

Weeks 3 to 4

- Discontinue use of sling
- Use immobilizer for sleep ** to be discontinued at 4 weeks unless otherwise directed by physician
- Continue gentle ROM exercises (PROM and AAROM)
  - Flexion to 90 degrees
  - Abduction to 90 degrees
  - ER/IR at 45 degrees and in scapular plane
  - ER in scapular plane to 15 to 20 degrees
  - IR in scapular plane to 55 to 60 degrees
  - **NOTE: Rate of progression based on evaluation of the patient
- No excessive ER, extension or elevation
- Continue isometrics and rhythmic stabilization (submax on land or pool)

Pool therapy
- Bouyancy-assisted flexion to 90 degrees (elbow extended)
- Prone hang to 90 degrees
- ER/IR movements
- Arm circles
- Pendulums
- Scapular strengthening patterns
- Core stabilization program
- Initiate scapular strengthening program
- Pool to include scapula squeezes, ER/IR AROM (avoid excessive ER)
- Continue use of cryotherapy

Weeks 5 to 6

- Gradually improve ROM
  - Flexion to 145 degrees
  - ER at 45 degrees abduction: 55 to 50 degrees
  - IR at 45 degrees abduction: 55 to 60 degrees
- May initiate stretching exercises
- Initiate exercise tubing ER/IR (arm at side) (land and pool)
- Scapular strengthening
- PNF manual resistance, water resistance
- Pool Exercises: AROM full can, abduction, ER/IR, scapular rowing, horizontal abd/adduction

II. Phase II: Intermediate Phase—Moderate Protection Phase (Weeks 7 to 14)

Goals:
- Gradually restore full ROM (week 10)
- Preserve the integrity of the surgical repair
- Restore muscular strength and balance
- Enhance neuromuscular control

Weeks 7 to 9

- Gradually progress ROM
  - Flexion to 160 degrees
  - Initiate ER/IR at 90 degrees abd
  - ER at 90 degrees abduction: 70 to 80 degrees at week 7
  - ER to 90 degrees at weeks 8 to 9
  - IR at 90 degrees abduction: 70 to 75 degrees
- Continue to progress isotonic strengthening program
- Continue PNF strengthening
- Pool Exercises: Initiate resisted ER/IR, scaption, scapula stabs with paddles

Weeks 10 to 14

- May initiate slightly more aggressive strengthening
- Progress isotonic strengthening exercises
- Continue all stretching exercises
  **Progress ROM to functional demands (ie, overhead athlete)
- Progress to isotonic strengthening (light and restricted ROM)
- Pool Exercises: PNF patterns, resistance paddles, functional movements, prone push with paddles, push ups

III. Phase III—Minimal Protection Phase (Weeks 15 to 20)

Goals:
- Maintain full ROM
- Improve muscular strength, power, and endurance
- Gradually initiate functional activities

Criteria to enter phase III:

1. Full, non-painful ROM
2. Satisfactory stability
3. Muscular strength (good grade or better)
4. No pain or tenderness

Weeks 15 to 18

- Continue all stretching exercises (capsular stretches)
- Continue strengthening exercises:
  - Throwers ten program or fundamental exercises
  - PNF manual resistance
  - Endurance training
  - Restricted sport activities (light swimming, half golf swings)
  - Pool: consider sport-specific motions
  - Initiate interval sport program weeks 16 to 18

Weeks 18 to 20

- Continue all exercise listed above
- Process interval sport program (throwing, etc)

IV. Phase IV—Advanced Strengthening Phase (Weeks 21 to 24)

Goals:

- Enhance muscular strength, power, and endurance
- Progress functional activities
- Maintain shoulder mobility

Criteria to Enter Phase IV:

1. Full, non-painful ROM
2. Satisfactory static stability
3. Muscular strength 75% to 80% of contralateral side
4. No pain or tenderness

Weeks 21 to 24

- Continue flexibility exercises
- Continue isotonic strengthening program
- NM control drills
- Plyometric strengthening
- Progress interval sport programs

V. Phase V—Return to Activity Phase (Months 7 to 9)

Goals:

- Gradual return to sport activities
- Maintain strength, mobility, and stability

Criteria to Enter Phase V:

1. Full functional ROM
2. Satisfactory isokinetic test that fulfills criteria
3. Satisfactory shoulder stability
4. No pain or tenderness

Exercises:

- Gradually progress sport activities to unrestrictive participation
- Continue stretching and strengthening program

KEW/JRA/LM:7/11

Appendix G

Rehabilitation Following Arthroscopic Rotator Cuff Repair—Small to Medium Tears

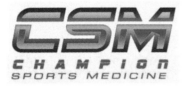

I. Phase I—Immediate Post-Surgical Phase (Days 1 to 10)

Goals:
- Maintain integrity of the repair
- Gradually increase passive range of motion
- Diminish pain and inflammation
- Prevent muscular inhibition

Days 1 to 6:
- Abduction pillow brace
- Pendulum exercises
- Active assisted range of motion (ROM) exercise (L-Bar)
  - ER/IR in scapular plane at 45 degrees of abduction (pain-free ROM)
  - Passive ROM
    - Flexion to tolerance (painful ROM)
    - ER/IR in scapular plane at 45 degrees of abduction (pain-free ROM)
- Elbow/hand gripping and ROM exercises
- Submaximal pain-free isometrics (initiate days 4 to 5)
  - Flexion with elbow bent to 90 degrees
  - External rotation
  - Internal rotation
  - Elbow flexors
- Cryotherapy for pain and inflammation
  - Ice 15 to 20 minutes every hour
- Sleeping
  - Sleep in pillow brace

Wilk KE, Joyner DM. *The Use of Aquatics in Orthopedic and Sports Medicine Rehabilitation and Physical Conditioning (pp 157-162).*
© 2014 SLACK Incorporated.

Days 7 to 10:

- Continue use of pillow brace
- Pendulum exercises
- Progress passive ROM to tolerance
  - Flexion to at least 115 degrees
  - ER in scapular plane at 45 degrees abduction to 20 to 25 degrees
  - IR in scapular plane at 45 degrees abduction to 30 to 35 degrees
- Active assisted ROM exercises (L-bar)
  - ER/IR in scapular plane at 45 degrees abduction
  - Flexion to tolerance*

    *Therapist provides assistance by supporting arm (especially with arm lowering)
- Continue elbow/hand ROM and gripping exercises
- Continue isometrics (submaximal and subpainful)
  - Flexion with bent elbow
  - Extension with bent elbow
  - Abduction with bent elbow
  - ER/IR with arm in scapular plane
  - Elbow flexion
- Initiate rhythmic stabilization ER/IR at 45 degrees abduction
- Continue use of ice for pain control
  - Use ice at least 6 to 7 times daily
- Sleeping
  - Continue sleeping in brace until physician instructs

Precautions:
1. No lifting of objects
2. No excessive shoulder extension
3. No excessive stretching or sudden movements
4. No supporting of body weight by hands
5. Keep incision clean and dry

II. Phase II—Protection Phase (Day 15 to Week 6)

Goals:
- Allow healing of soft tissue
- Do not overstress healing tissue
- Gradually restore full passive ROM (Weeks 4 to 5)
- Re-establish dynamic shoulder stability
- Decrease pain and inflammation

Days 15 to 21:

- Continue use of sling or brace (physician or therapist will determine when to discontinue)
- Passive ROM to tolerance
  - Flexion to 140 to 155 degrees
  - ER at 90 degrees abduction to at least 45 degrees
  - IR at 90 degrees abduction to at least 45 degrees
- Active assisted ROM to tolerance
  - Flexion (continue use of arm support)
  - ER/IR in scapular plane at 45 degrees abduction
  - ER/IR at 90 degrees abduction
  - Buoyancy-assisted flexion in pool (once wounds are healed; initiate with elbow straight)
- Dynamic stabilization drills
  - Rhythmic stabilization drills
    - ER/IR in scapular plane
    - Flexion/extension at 100 degrees flexion and 125 degrees flexion
- Continue all isometric contractions (land and pool)
- Initiate scapular isometrics
- Continue use of cryotherapy as needed
- Continue all precautions
  - No lifting
  - No excessive motion

Weeks 4 to 5:

- Patient should exhibit full passive range of motion by week 4
- Continue all exercises listed above
- Initiate ER/IR strengthening using exercise tubing at 0 degrees of abduction (use towel roll)
- Pool exercises: AROM ER/IR in pool, pendulums, arm circles
- Initiate manual resistance ER supine in scapular plane (light resistance)
- Initiate prone rowing to neutral arm position (land and pool)
- Initiate prone shoulder extension (land and pool)
- Initiate ER strengthening exercises
- Initiate isotonic elbow flexion
- Continue use of ice as needed
- May use heat prior to ROM exercises
- Pool exercises; May use pool for light AROM exercises
- Rhythmic stabilization exercises (flexion 45, 90, 125 degrees; ER/IR)

Weeks 5 to 6:

- May use heat prior to exercises
- Continue AAROM and stretching exercises
  - Especially for movements that are not full
    - Shoulder flexion
    - ER at 90 degrees abduction
    - Supine in pool to work on end range flexion
- Initiate active ROM exercises
  - Shoulder flexion scapular plane (consider pool if + shrug)
  - Shoulder abduction
- Progress isotonic strengthening exercise program
  - ER tubing
  - Sidelying ER
  - Prone rowing
  - Prone horizontal abduction (bent elbow)
  - Biceps curls (isotonics)
  - Pool exercises: small paddles to increase resistance in the pool during ER/IR and arm circles, initiate horizontal movements

Precautions:

1. No heavy lifting of objects
2. No excessive behind the back movements
3. No supporting of body weight by hands and arms
4. No sudden jerking motions

III. Phase III—Intermediate Phase (Weeks 7 to 14)

Goals:
- Full active ROM (Weeks 8 to 10)
- Maintain full passive ROM
- Dynamic shoulder stability
- Gradual restoration of shoulder strength
- Gradual return to functional activities

Week 7:

- Continue stretching and PROM (as needed to maintain full ROM)
- Continue dynamic stabilization drills
- Progress strengthening program
  - ER/IR tubing
  - ER sidelying
  - Lateral raises*
  - Full can in scapular plane*
  - Prone rowing

- ○ Prone horizontal abduction
- ○ Prone extension
- ○ Elbow flexion
- ○ Elbow extension
- ○ Pool exercises: initiate larger resistance paddles if appropriate

*Patient must be able to elevate arm without shoulder or scapular hiking before initiating isotonics; if unable, continue glenohumeral joint exercises.

Week 8:

- Continue all exercise listed above
- If physician permits, may initiate light functional activities

Week 10:

- Continue all exercise listed above
- Progress to fundamental shoulder exercises
- Therapist may initiate isotonic resistance (1 Ib weight) during flexion and abduction*
  - ○ *If non-painful normal motion is exhibited!

Weeks 11 to 14:

- Progress all exercises
  - ○ Continue ROM and flexibility exercises
  - ○ Progress strengthening program (increase 1 Ib/10 days *non-painful)
  - ○ Pool exercises: functional movements in pool- PNF, overhead reach in prone

IV. Phase IV—Advanced Strengthening Phase (Weeks 15 to 22)

Goals:
- Maintain full non-painful ROM
- Enhance functional use of upper extremity
- Improve muscular strengthen and power
- Gradual return to functional activities

Week 15:

- Continue ROM and stretching to maintain full ROM
- Self capsular stretches
- Progress shoulder strengthening exercises
  - ○ Fundamental shoulder exercises
- Initiate interval golf program (if appropriate)
- Baseball, golf, tennis swing in pool

Weeks 20 to 22:

- Continue all exercises listed above
- Progress golf program to playing golf (if appropriate)

- Initiate interval tennis program (if appropriate)
- May initiate swimming (if appropriate); physician must clear

V. Phase V—Return to Activity Phase (Weeks 23 to 36)

Goals:
- Gradual return to strenuous work activities
- Gradual return to recreational sport activities

Week 23:

- Continue fundamental shoulder exercise program (at least 4 times weekly)
- Continue stretching, if motion is tight
- Continue progression to sport participation

KWJA 4/07

Appendix H

Arthroscopic Slap Lesion Repair (Type II)

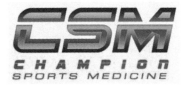

I. Phase I—Immediate Postoperative Phase "Restrictive Motion" (Day 1 to Week 6)

Goals:

- Protect the anatomic repair
- Prevent negative effects of immobilization
- Promote dynamic stability
- Diminish pain and inflammation

Weeks 0 to 2:

- Sling for 4 weeks
- Sleep in immobilizer for 4 weeks
- Elbow/hand range of motion (ROM)
- Hand gripping exercises
- Passive and gentle active assistive ROM exercise
  - Flexion to 60 degrees (Week 2: flexion to 75 degrees)
  - Elevation in scapular plane to 60 degrees
  - ER/IR with arm in scapular plane
  - ER to 10 to 15 degrees
  - IR to 45 degrees
  - **NO active ER or extension or abduction
- Submaximal isometrics for shoulder musculature
- NO isolated biceps contractions
- Cryotherapy, modalities as indicated

Weeks 3 to 4:

- Discontinue use of sling at 4 weeks
- Sleep in immobilizer until Week 4

Wilk KE, Joyner DM. *The Use of Aquatics in Orthopedic and Sports Medicine Rehabilitation and Physical Conditioning (pp 163-166).*
© 2014 SLACK Incorporated.

- Continue gentle ROM exercises (PROM and AAROM)
  - Flexion to 90 degrees
  - Abduction to 75 to 85 degrees
  - ER in scapular plane and 35 degrees abd to 25 to 30 degrees
  - IR in scapular plane and 35 degrees abd to 55 to 60 degrees
  - **NOTE: Rate of progression based on evaluation of the patient.
- No active ER, extension, or elevation
- Initiate rhythmic stabilization drills
- Initiate proprioception training
- Tubing ER/IR at 0 degrees abduction
- Continue isometrics (land and pool)
- Pool exercises: AAROM to 90 degrees, ER/IR at side (avoid excessive motions), arm circles, pendulums, rowing movements
  - Prone and standing AROM in pool
- Continue use of cryotherapy

Weeks 5 to 6:

- Gradually improve ROM
  - Flexion to 145 degrees
  - ER at 45 degrees abduction: 45 to 50 degrees
  - ER at 45 degrees abduction: 55 to 60 degrees
  - At 6 weeks begin light and gradual ER at 90 degree abduction – progress to 30 to 40 degrees ER
- May initiate stretching exercises (supine and prone in pool)
- May initiate light (easy) ROM at 90 degrees abduction
- Continue tubing ER/IR (arm at side)
- PNF manual resistance (AROM in pool)
- Initiate active shoulder abduction (without resistance)
- Initiate "full can" exercise (weight of arm)
- Initiate prone rowing, prone horizontal abduction
- Pool exercises: AROM in pool- (standing and prone for abduction and scaption; scapula)
- NO biceps strengthening

II. Phase II—Intermediate Phase: Moderate Protection Phase (Weeks 7 to 14)

Goals:
- Gradually restore full ROM (Week 10)
- Preserve the integrity of the surgical repair
- Restore muscular strength and balance

Weeks 7 to 9:

- Gradually progress ROM:
  - Flexion to 180 degrees
  - ER at 90 degrees abduction: 90 to 95 degrees

- IR at 90 degrees abduction: 70 to 75 degrees
- Continue to progress isotonic strengthening program
- Continue PNF strengthening
- Initiate throwers ten program
- Pool exercises: small paddles to increase resistance during ER/IR and shoulder and scapular movement patterns

Weeks 10 to 12:

- May initiate slightly more aggressive strengthening
- Progress ER to throwers motion
  - ER at 90 degrees abduction: 110 to 115 in throwers (Weeks 10 to 12)
- Progress isotonic strengthening exercises
- Continue all stretching exercises

**Progress ROM to functional demands (ie, overhead athlete)

- Continue all strengthening exercises
- Pool exercises: progress paddle sizes in pool, functional movements, PNF, push/pull, etc

III. Phase III—Minimal Protection Phase (Weeks 14 to 20)

Goals:
- Establish and maintain full ROM
- Improve muscular strength, power and endurance
- Gradually initiate functional activities

Criteria to enter Phase III:
1. Full non-painful ROM
2. Satisfactory stability
3. Muscular strength (good grade or better)
4. No pain or tenderness

Weeks 14 to 16:

- Continue all stretching exercises (capsular stretches)
- Maintain throwers motion (Especially ER)
- Continue strengthening exercises:
  - Throwers ten program or fundamental exercises
  - PNF manual resistance
  - Endurance training
  - Initiate light plyometric program
  - Restricted sport activities (light swimming, half golf swings)
  - Pool exercises: golf, tennis, baseball swing; progressive strengthening
  - Pool exercises: prone pushes in pool with flotation devices

Weeks 16 to 20:

- Continue all exercise listed above
- Continue all stretching

- Continue throwers ten program
- Progress pool program with larger paddles, swimming (limited swim style); physician must clear
- Continue plyometric program
- Initiate interval sport program (throwing, etc)

**See interval throwing program

IV. Phase IV—Advanced Strengthening Phase (Weeks 20 to 26)

Goals:
- Enhanced muscular strength, power and endurance
- Progress functional activities
- Maintain shoulder mobility

Criteria to enter Phase IV:
1. Full, non-painful ROM
2. Satisfactory static stability
3. Muscular strength 75% to 80% of contralateral side
4. No pain or tenderness

Weeks 20 to 26:

- Continue flexibility exercises
- Continue isotonic strengthening program
- PNF manual resistance patterns
- Plyometric strengthening
- Progress interval sport programs

V. Phase V—Return to Activity Phase (Months 6 to 9)

Goals:
- Gradual return to sport activities
- Maintain strength, mobility and stability

Criteria to enter Phase V:
1. Full functional ROM
2. Muscular performance isokinetic (fulfills criteria)
3. Satisfactory shoulder stability
4. No pain or tenderness

Exercises:
- Gradually progress sport activities to unrestrictive participation
- Continue stretching and strengthening program

KEW/JRA/LM: 7/11

Appendix I

Lumbar Stabilization Aquatic Therapy Protocol

PHASE I

Goals:

- Diminish inflammation, swelling, and pain
- Centralize radicular symptoms
- Reduce muscle spasm
- Restore 75% of normal range of motion (ROM) (especially lumbar extension)
- Restore voluntary core stabilization muscle activation
- Pain = 5/10
- Prevent dysfunction of extremities due to compensations
- Provide patient education on anatomy and lumbar function

Weight Bearing: As tolerated

Aquatic Exercises:

- Standing back bends to tolerance
- TA isometrics – sitting and/or standing
- Slow TM ambulation with UE ||-bar support
- Slow rotations (standing) with forearms on a kick board
- Lx neutral, back against wall shallow squats
- HS, quads, gastrocs, piriformis, iliopsoas stretches
- Supported floating; UE/LE AROM

Aqua Massager: Massage sore/spasmed Lx muscles and along the sciatic nerve tract to tolerance if radicular symptoms exist.

Patient Education: Educate on extension and neutral stabilization principles. Teach proper sitting and standing posture. Practice safe transfers with emphasis on protection of unstable or painful lumbar region.

PHASE II

Goals:

- Restore full lumbar ROM
- Pain = 3/10
- Minimal muscle spasm
- Core muscle isometric holds with UE/LE movement

Wilk KE, Joyner DM. *The Use of Aquatics in Orthopedic and Sports Medicine Rehabilitation and Physical Conditioning (pp 167–168)*.
© 2014 SLACK Incorporated.

- Slow gait without compensations

Aquatic Exercises:
- Standing back bends
- TA Isometrics with UE movements in sagittal/frontal/transverse planes
- TA Isometrics with LE movements in sagittal/frontal/transverse planes
- TM ambulation 75% of normal speed with UE ||-bar support
- TM ambulation 50% of normal speed without UE support
- Squats with UE support
- Lunges in sagittal and frontal planes
- Continue LE stretching program
- Semi-supported floating

Aqua Massager: Continue use on sore/spasmed muscles.

Education: Emphasis on safe progression of exercise and plan for return to normal activities and work.

Phase III

Goals:
- Minimal pain
- No muscle spasm
- Core muscle contraction with functional movements
- Normal gait
- Move at functional rate
- Return to all functional and work activities

Aquatic Exercises:
- Deep squats with resistance and versus jets in 3-planes
- TM ambulation at faster than normal speed
- Resisted UE exercise (using hydrobells) with Lx neutral
  - single and bilateral
  - increase pace
- 3-plane lunges with UE resistance
- Single LE stance activities
  - with UE resistance
  - versus jets
- Simulate ADLs and work activities
- Continue LE stretching program

Aqua Massager: As needed in areas of spasm, discomfort, pain

Education: Ergonomics and body mechanics for specific daily activities and work functions. Emphasis should be on efficient movement and prevention of future injuries.

Reprinted with permission from Timothy DiFrancesco, PT, DPT, ATC, CSCS, AQx, CMT.

APPENDIX J

Herniated Discs and Degenerative Joint Disease Protocol

Level 1: Weeks 1 to 3

Introduce the below exercises for 1 to 3 sets of 20-second holds. Progress to 1 to 3 sets of 90- to 120-second holds by adding 10 to 15 seconds each session.

- Anti-extension
  - Superman
- Anti-rotation
  - C.A.R.P with tubing

Level 2: Weeks 4 to 6

Introduce the below exercises for 1 to 3 sets of 6 to 8 reps. Progress to 1 to 3 sets of 8 to 15 reps.

- Hip extension
  - CSD with noodle
- Hip ABD/ADD
  - CSD with abd/add

Level 3: Weeks 7 to 12

Introduce the below exercises for 1 to 3 sets of 6 to 8 reps. Progress to 1 to 3 sets of 8 to 15 reps.

- Squat/dead-lift variations
  - Overhead squat
  - DL with wall reach
  - Swing with DB (one hand/two hand)
- Step ups
  - Linear to box
  - Linear to box with medicine ball
  - Lateral to box
  - Lateral to box with medicine ball
- Lunge series
  - Linear to box
  - Retro from box
  - Linear to box with medicine ball
  - Retro from box with medicine ball

Wilk KE, Joyner DM. *The Use of Aquatics in Orthopedic and Sports Medicine Rehabilitation and Physical Conditioning* (pp 169-171).
© 2014 SLACK Incorporated.

Protocol for: Spinal Stenosis/Stress Reaction, Stress Fracture, Spondylolysis/ Spondylolisthesis/Traumatic Injuries to the Cervical, Thoracic, or Lumbar Spine/ Compression Fracture With and Without Vertebroplasty/ Scoliosis

Level 1: Weeks 1 to 3

Introduce the below exercise for 1 to 3 sets of 20-second holds. Progress to 1 to 3 sets of 90- to 120-second holds by adding 10 to 15 seconds each session.

- Anti-rotation
  - C.A.R.P with tubing

Introduce the below exercises for 1 to 3 sets of 10 reps. Progress to 1 to 3 sets of 20 reps.

- Shallow water primitive patterns
  - Quadruped belly breathing
  - Quadruped glute ext
  - Quadruped glute abdextension

Level 2: Weeks 4 to 6

Introduce the below exercises for 1 to 3 sets of 6 to 8 reps. Progress to 1 to 3 sets of 8 to 15 reps.

- Hip extension
  - CSD with noodle
- Hip ABD/ADD
  - CSD with abd/add

Level 3: Weeks 7 to 9

Introduce the below exercises for 1 to 3 sets of 6 to 8 reps. Progress to 1 to 3 sets of 8 to 15 reps.

- Step ups
  - Linear to box
  - Linear to box with medicine ball
  - Lateral to box
  - Lateral to box with medicine ball
- Lunge series
  - Linear to box
  - Retro from box
  - Linear to box with medicine ball
  - Retro from box with medicine ball

Level 4: Weeks 9 to 12

Introduce the below exercises for 1 to 3 sets of 6 to 8 reps. Progress to 1 to 3 sets of 8 to 15 reps.

- Hip hinge with kick board
- Squat/dead-lift variations
  - Overhead squat
  - DL with wall reach
  - Swing with DB (one hand/two hand)
  - Squat with row/pull back

Introduce the below exercise for 1 to 3 sets of 20-second holds. Progress to 1 to 3 sets of 90- to 120-second holds by adding 10 to 15 seconds each session.

- Stair side plank
  - Buoyancy supported

Financial Disclosures

Dr. James R. Andrews has not disclosed any relevant financial relationships.

Dr. Bruce E. Becker has not disclosed any relevant financial relationships.

Dr. Stephen F. Crouse received research grant and equipment provided to Texas A&M University, specifically for his laboratory to conduct scientific research on exercise equipment manufactured by HydroWorx International, Inc. He also received consulting fees paid by HydroWorx International, Inc for speaking at sponsored workshops and conferences.

Dr. Timothy DiFrancesco has no financial or proprietary interest in the materials presented herein.

Dr. Dennis Dolny has no financial or proprietary interest in the materials presented herein.

Mr. Anson J. Flake has no financial or proprietary interest in the materials presented herein.

Mr. Murphy Grant has not disclosed any relevant financial relationships.

Ms. Jessica Heath has not disclosed any relevant financial relationships.

Dr. Todd R. Hooks has not disclosed any relevant financial relationships.

Dr. David M. Joyner has not disclosed any relevant financial relationships.

Mr. Leonard C. Macrina has no financial or proprietary interest in the materials presented herein.

Mr. Jason Palmer has no financial or proprietary interest in the materials presented herein.

Dr. Lisa Pataky has no financial or proprietary interest in the materials presented herein.

Dr. Mike Reinold has not disclosed any relevant financial relationships.

Mr. Daniel Seidler has not disclosed any relevant financial relationships.

Dr. Kevin E. Wilk has not disclosed any relevant financial relationships.

Dr. A. J. Yenchak has no financial or proprietary interest in the materials presented herein.

INDEX